# PREVENTING MATERNAL DEATHS

Edited by

**Erica Royston**
Division of Family Health
World Health Organization
Geneva, Switzerland

&

**Sue Armstrong**
Freelance journalist
London, England

WORLD HEALTH ORGANIZATION
GENEVA
1989

ISBN 92 4 156128 9

TYPESET IN INDIA
PRINTED IN ENGLAND
88/7817—Macmillans/Clays—7000

# CONTENTS

Contents

Chapter 9
**The role of family planning in preventing maternal deaths**

Chapter 10
**The challenge**

# CONTRIBUTORS

While the final text of this book is a synthesis of countless experiences and insights, ten people wrote original drafts for individual chapters. The process of moulding the themes into a coherent whole, and the enrichment resulting from the collaboration of so many enthusiastic and knowledgeable individuals, have substantially changed much of the original text—to such an extent that each of the chapters is now the work of several people. For this reason, we have preferred not to attribute individual chapters to those who wrote the first drafts, but simply to list here the contributors:

Sue Armstrong, Freelance journalist, London, England;
Kathy Canavan, Yale University School of Medicine, New Haven, CT, USA;
Robert Cook, Division of Family Health, WHO, Geneva, Switzerland;
Kelsey Harrison, University of Port Harcourt, Nigeria;
Sarah Lewitt, Population Council, New York, USA;
Alan Lopez, Division of Epidemiological Surveillance and Health Situation and Trend Assessment, WHO, Geneva, Switzerland;
Erica Royston, Division of Family Health, WHO, Geneva, Switzerland;
Beatrice Selwyn, University of Texas, Houston, TX, USA;
Christopher Tietze, Population Council, New York, USA (sadly, Dr Tietze died during the preparation of this publication); and
Beverly Winikoff, Population Council, New York, USA.

# ACKNOWLEDGEMENTS

Many people have been involved in the preparation of this monograph since its inception in 1983, and we should like to express our gratitude to all of them for their efforts, enthusiasm and advice.

Very particular thanks are due to Angèle Petros-Barvazian for her support, encouragement and expert guidance throughout the development of this book; to Mark Belsey and Barbara Kwast for their detailed technical review and advice in this diverse field; to Vicki Hammer for her encouragement in the early days; to Deborah Howard and Jane Ferguson for their painstaking library work and help in establishing the data base; and to Janet Demierre, Jackie Haines, Lindsay Hernandez and June Mitchell for their invaluable secretarial back-up. In addition, we owe a fundamental debt of gratitude to the countless researchers in the field whose information, and often fascinating insights, have been the bedrock of this monograph.

The generous financial contribution of the United Nations Population Fund to this project is also gratefully acknowledged.

# Chapter 1

# INTRODUCTION

---

Childbirth is a universally celebrated event, an occasion for dancing, fireworks, flowers or gifts. Yet, for many thousands of women each day, childbirth is experienced not as the joyful event it should be, but as a private hell that may end in death. In practically every society, celebration of life is the dominant theme, while the grimmer side of childbearing is often shrouded in silence, known only to those who suffer it and those who attend them.

In fact, maternal death and injury in developing countries constitute a tragedy of vast proportions. Yet it is a tragedy that has been largely ignored by those who set national and international health priorities, because those who suffer generally live in remote places, are poor, illiterate and politically powerless.

Today the rates of maternal mortality in rich and poor countries show a greater disparity than any other public health indicator—including the infant mortality rate, which is most often taken as the measure of comparative disadvantage. Thus, for a woman in the developing world, the average lifetime risk of dying of a pregnancy-related cause is between one in 15 and one in 50, compared with an average lifetime risk of between one in 4000 and one in 10 000 for a woman in the developed world.

This situation has existed for many years, but because childbearing is essentially a healthy and welcomed process, traditional societies have somehow accepted the risks as normal and unavoidable. It is only very recently that people have started to challenge—loudly and clearly in international forums—the stifling mix of personal fatalism and political disregard for women's needs that has condoned inaction in many poor countries.

Under the spotlight of the United Nations Decade for Women (1976–85), the sheer scale of the suffering associated with maternity became widely recognized. So, too, did the crucial fact that most of this suffering is preventable, and that Health for All by the Year 2000 is just an empty slogan if glaring inequities in health care provision are allowed to continue.

There are encouraging signs that people are now beginning to build on this new awareness, with practical commitment to maternal health at the national and international levels. It is the purpose of this book to encourage the initiative by pulling together in one place diverse reports and fragments of information on maternal mortality, and thereby to give an overview of current knowledge on this major public health problem.

The book is also intended to be a catalyst for change in public health policy by establishing the special and long-neglected health needs of women as a high priority.

Since the book is intended for a wide range of people concerned with women's health—from the general reader to the specialist seeking particular information on the causes of, and possible solutions to, maternal mortality—it has been necessary to cover both basic and more specialized information. We hope that readers will bear with the material that is not relevant to their personal inquiry.

Of great encouragement is the fact that the concerted international effort to lower the infant mortality rate in poor countries in recent years has been very successful in saving young lives. The same can be achieved in the field of maternal mortality. We have the knowledge to make childbearing safe; success depends now on broad public support and a strengthening of political will.

# Chapter 2

# MEASURING MATERNAL MORTALITY

## Definitions

### Maternal death

Intuitively one would expect the definition of a maternal
death to be a simple matter. Childbirth is a memorable event
and death in childbirth even more so. In practice, however,
matters are not so clear cut. If the definition of a maternal
death is to include all deaths due to pregnancy and childbirth it must include deaths taking place before childbirth
(e.g., due to abortion, ectopic pregnancy), those taking
place during childbirth (e.g., due to antepartum, intra-
partum or postpartum haemorrhage), as well as deaths taking
place some time after the actual event of childbirth (e.g.,
due to sepsis). Moreover, not all maternal deaths are directly
due to conditions resulting solely from pregnancy. Some are
caused by pre-existing conditions which are aggravated by
pregnancy (e.g., hepatitis). This latter distinction is not new.
Traditionally, maternal deaths have been classified as "true"
maternal deaths when the pregnancy was directly responsible
for the sequence of events that led to the death, and
"associated" or "indirect" where the condition that led to
the death was unrelated to the pregnancy (1). This distinction
is reiterated in the Ninth Revision of the International
Classification of Diseases (ICD-9), which defines a maternal
death as follows (2):

A maternal death is defined as the death of a woman while
pregnant or within 42 days of termination of pregnancy,
irrespective of the duration and the site of the pregnancy, from
any cause related to or aggravated by the pregnancy or its
management but not from accidental or incidental causes.

Maternal deaths should be subdivided into two groups:

(1) Direct obstetric deaths: those resulting from obstetric
complications of the pregnant state (pregnancy, labour and
puerperium), from interventions, omissions, incorrect treatment,
or from a chain of events resulting from any of the above.

11

(2) Indirect obstetric deaths: those resulting from previous existing disease or disease that developed during pregnancy and which was not due to direct obstetric causes, but which was aggravated by physiologic effects of pregnancy.

Implicit in this definition is the notion of exclusion—"a maternal death is the death of a woman while pregnant . . . but *not* from accidental or incidental causes"—which if followed could significantly reduce the bias inherent in most of the maternal mortality rates published today. A working group on health statistics, meeting in Geneva in 1974, preferred to use the following definition of a maternal death: "the death of a woman while pregnant or within 42 days of termination of pregnancy irrespective of the duration of or the site of the pregnancy". The group went on to say: "this should be the total definition. We wish to have included in 'maternal mortality' all known deaths of women known to be pregnant. In this regard all death certificates of women in the reproductive age group, 12–50, should have the certificate specially annotated if the woman was known to be pregnant at the time of her death or was known to have been pregnant at any time within the previous 42 days. Maternal death should then be subdivided into three groups: firstly, direct obstetric death, secondly, indirect obstetric death and, thirdly, the fortuitous or coincidental death of a woman where the condition causing the death was not obstetric and was not aggravated by the obstetric state. It is realized that in many situations it will not be possible to obtain information on all deaths in the three categories but certainly the principles should be maintained."[1] Maternal mortality is thus being defined as a 'time of death' measure, analogous to infant mortality, which can, where such information is available, also be analysed by cause.

The ratio between the three components of maternal mortality thus defined will depend critically on the level of maternal mortality. In countries where the level is low, the inclusion of external causes might render an estimate of maternal mortality less useful for monitoring and planning. Fortunately, these are usually countries with good cause-of-death registration, where the separation into the three components should not pose any insurmountable difficulties. In countries where the maternal mortality rate (MMR) is

---

[1] *Report of a working group on health statistics in relation to maternal health and perinatal events, Geneva, 12–16 September 1983.* Unpublished WHO document DES/ICD-10/83.10.

high, the bias introduced into estimates of maternal mortality by the inclusion of external causes is usually very low and well worth the overall improvement in the total estimate. In rural Bangladesh (MMR = 570 per 100 000 births) it was found, for example, that 90% of deaths of women who were pregnant, or had been pregnant within the preceding 90 days, were due to maternal causes (3). An Egyptian inquiry (MMR = 263 per 100 000 births) found 87% of such deaths to be due to maternal causes (4).

## Maternal mortality rate

While the number of maternal deaths occurring in a given locality (or country) is a useful measure of magnitude and can be used for the planning of maternal and child health (MCH) services or for the analysis of causes, it cannot be used as an indicator to measure change or to make comparisons between locations. Moreover, the total number of maternal deaths is a function of two variables—fertility, i.e., the probability of becoming pregnant and, once pregnant, the risk of dying from maternal causes. A reduction in either component can effect a reduction in the proportion of women dying from maternal causes. (The enormous differentials in maternal mortality rates in the world thus tell only half the story.)

The maternal mortality rate, the most commonly used indicator of maternal death, measures a woman's chances of dying from a given pregnancy and should, theoretically, relate the number of maternal deaths (as the numerator) to the total number of pregnancies (as the denominator). Ideally, therefore, the numerator should include all deaths defined as "maternal deaths" in a given time interval, and the denominator all episodes of pregnancy occurring in the same time interval, regardless of their outcome.

In practice, however, neither concept can be generally employed. Even in countries with the most advanced and efficient vital registration systems, women whose pregnancy results in a spontaneous abortion any time during the first 28 weeks are not registered and hence are automatically excluded from the population at risk of dying from a maternal death (although they may appear in the numerator if the cause of death is diagnosed as such). Similarly, the recording of pregnancies that result in a late fetal death is often far from complete. As a result, the population at risk of maternal death is generally taken as the number of live births, which is assumed to be a good proxy indicator of the number of pregnancies. Typically, in countries with low induced abortion rates, the former is within 10% of the latter, which is unlikely to affect markedly the overall rate.

## How reliable are official rates?

Most official maternal mortality rates, with the notable exception of hospital rates, are underestimates. The reasons for this will vary according to certification practices, the degree of sophistication of the vital registration system or whether indeed a vital registration system exists at all. The UN estimates that vital registration of death data exists in 69 of the 166 Member States of WHO, covering a total population of 1452 million, or about 30% of the world's population (5).

Where good vital registration does exist, the biases are usually due to incorrect classification of the cause of death. There may be many social, religious, emotional or practical reasons for not classifying a maternal death as such. Deaths of unmarried women or those resulting from the complications of abortion, for example, may often be classified under another cause to avoid embarrassing the surviving family; this is all the more likely if the abortion was illegal. The extent of this type of under-reporting can be considerable. Another common cause for under-reporting is a wish to avoid blame.

In most developed countries and in most hospital settings all over the world there is usually an inquiry following a maternal death. It is, therefore, not difficult to imagine that in many cultures this constitutes a strong incentive to attribute a maternal death to a less blameworthy cause. Such misrepresentation may not be very common in countries with a tradition of "no name, no blame" confidential inquiries, but seems to be quite common elsewhere. (In such situations the instigation of a system of confidential inquiries may, in fact, be counterproductive.)

In countries with very low rates of maternal mortality, very few maternal deaths actually take place in obstetric departments of large hospitals because, when life-threatening conditions, such as acute renal failure, arise the patient is usually transferred to another specialist department. If she dies there the death will be certified by a non-obstetric specialist and the cause of death appearing on the certificate may well not mention the obstetric condition which triggered the fatal sequence of events.

Evidently, even in countries where all or most deaths are medically certified, maternity-related mortality can still be grossly underestimated. A study conducted in the USA by the New Jersey Health Department identified an additional 26 maternal deaths in that State during 1974–75 over and above the 30 deaths reported in the vital statistics (6). A study carried out by the Centers for Disease Control found that the incidence of maternal mortality in the USA in 1974–78 was 12.1 per 100 000 live births rather than the reported rate of 9.6 (7). Intensive surveillance through a review of death certificates and selected medical records in Puerto Rico in 1978 and 1979 revealed that only about 27% of pregnancy-related deaths had been recorded through the registration system.[1] By linking death certificates of women in the childbearing ages with birth certificates of their offspring, researchers reported a 50% increase in the number of known maternal deaths in Georgia in 1975 and 1976 compared with the figure obtained from vital registration (8).

It is clear that even in the most favourable circumstances, as in developed countries, and certainly in the far less favourable circumstances of most of the developing world, special efforts have to be made—and additional costs incurred—in order to get good data on maternal mortality. Whether the additional costs and efforts are worth while will depend on the uses to which the data are put. In general, the more precise the information the greater the cost, and it may well be that in order to plan and implement inter-ventions aimed at improving women's health a broad order of magnitude suffices.

Moreover, in most developed countries, a maternal death is a very rare event and is no longer a good indicator of the risks to women's health that result from their reproductive functions. A more holistic view of the reproductive health of women in these circumstances must include the risks that women run in order *not* to get pregnant, i.e., the risks of death resulting from contraceptive use. This notion has given rise to the development of what is called the *reproductive mortality rate* which includes not only pregnancy-related

---

[1] *Methodology for intensive surveillance of pregnancy-related deaths, Puerto Rico, 1978–1979.* Unpublished document of United States Department of Health, Education and Welfare, Center for Disease Control, Atlanta, GA.

deaths but also deaths from the side-effects of contraceptive methods. The latter can be estimated from data on the prevalence of oral contraception, use of intrauterine devices (IUDs) and sterilization, and from estimates of mortality risk associated with their use derived from epidemiological studies. An appropriate denominator in this case for approximating the person–years of exposure to risk would be the number of sexually active women in the reproductive age group. As this figure is not generally available, the total number of women in this age group is used instead. Whereas in 1955, 99% of the reproductive deaths in the United States were pregnancy-related, only slightly more than one-half (53%) were so in 1975. Virtually all of the remainder (45%) were related to oral contraceptive use (9). By way of contrast, in Menoufia, Egypt, in 1981–83 and in Bali, Indonesia, in 1980–82, 98% of reproductive mortality was pregnancy-related (10).

Intermediate between countries with good vital registration and those where there is incomplete or no coverage[1] of registration, there are many countries where the registration of deaths is fairly complete but registration of the cause of death is poor. Maternal mortality rates based on data derived from such systems can be extremely misleading. An indication of the degree of incompleteness of cause-of-death certification can be gleaned from the number of deaths classified as being due to "symptoms and ill-defined causes". In Thailand, for example, out of the 18 985 deaths of women aged 15–44 years registered in 1981, 863, or 5%, were registered as being from maternal causes, giving a maternal mortality rate of 81.2 per 100 000 births. However, an additional 6061 women, or 32%, died from "symptoms and ill-defined causes". Bearing in mind the problems of definition described above, one can safely guess that at least an equivalent proportion (i.e., at least 5% of 6061, or 300) also died from maternal causes, bringing the maternal mortality rate up to at least 109 per 100 000 births. If *all* the 6061 deaths from ill-defined causes were maternal, the maternal mortality rate would be 651, which is clearly an overestimate but is indicative of the degree of confidence that the "official" maternal mortality rate can inspire. As can be seen from Table 2.1, Thailand is far from being unique in this respect—in some countries as many as 63% of women's deaths are without specified cause.

---

[1] *Coverage*—the extent to which all population segments or subgroups are included in the registration system within a country; *completeness*—the extent to which all relevant events are counted.

Table 2.1. Maternal mortality rates, as reported and corrected for under-registration of cause of death (selected countries, 1970–1981)

| Country or area | Year | Maternal deaths per 100 000 live births | Proportion of deaths from ill-defined conditions in women aged 15–44 years % | 'Corrected' maternal deaths per 100 000 live births[a] | Difference due to correction % |
|---|---|---|---|---|---|
| Syrian Arab Republic | 1981 | 8 | 63 | 21 | 163 |
| Thailand | 1981 | 80 | 32 | 117 | 46 |
| El Salvador | 1974 | 95 | 28 | 133 | 40 |
| Honduras | 1979 | 82 | 28 | 106 | 29 |
| Nicaragua | 1978 | 65 | 25 | 87 | 34 |
| Dominican Republic | 1978 | 55 | 24 | 72 | 31 |
| Paraguay | 1980 | 469 | 16 | 555 | 18 |
| Guatemala | 1980 | 96 | 16 | 113 | 18 |
| Ecuador | 1978 | 216 | 14 | 250 | 16 |
| Guadeloupe | 1974 | 250 | 13 | 286 | 14 |
| Mauritius | 1980 | 108 | 12 | 122 | 13 |
| Guyana | 1977 | 104 | 11 | 117 | 13 |
| Suriname | 1980 | 82 | 11 | 91 | 11 |
| Fiji | 1978 | 53 | 11 | 58 | 9 |
| Mexico | 1976 | 119 | 10 | 131 | 10 |
| Sri Lanka | 1977 | 98 | 9 | 107 | 9 |
| Egypt | 1979 | 78 | 9 | 85 | 9 |
| Costa Rica | 1980 | 23 | 8 | 25 | 9 |
| Colombia | 1977 | 134 | 7 | 143 | 7 |
| Barbados | 1980 | 24 | 7 | 25 | 4 |
| Peru | 1977 | 172 | 7 | 185 | 8 |
| Philippines | 1977 | 142 | 7 | 152 | 7 |
| Chile | 1980 | 73 | 7 | 78 | 7 |
| Uruguay | 1977 | 82 | 3 | 84 | 2 |
| Argentina | 1979 | 78 | 5 | 82 | 6 |
| Trinidad and Tobago | 1977 | 82 | 3 | 84 | 2 |

[a] Rate based on deaths certified as maternal plus a proportion of the deaths of women of reproductive age that have been classified as being due to "symptoms and ill-defined causes" equal to the proportion of all deaths of women of reproductive age certified as maternal.

*Source*: World Health Organization. Data reported by Member States.

In areas where health care is largely provided by primary health care workers who do not have the necessary medical qualifications to certify deaths according to the sophisticated categories of the ICD, an alternative system of cause-of-death certification has to be used. WHO has developed a framework of classification based on lay reporting of symptoms on which health personnel can build and which can be used for classifying causes of death (*11*).

17

# Alternative ways of measuring maternal mortality

Only one-third of the world's population lives in countries
where the registration of births and deaths is fairly complete
and the certification of cause of death is reasonably reliable.
In other situations, where civil registration is incomplete or
nonexistent, other sources of information and other methods
have to be used. A variety of approaches have been tried,
with varying success; some of them are described below. Each
method has its advantages and its drawbacks and not all
approaches are feasible in all settings. It is possible to
visualize a hierarchy of situations depending on the sort of
records available and the degree of contact of the health
system or other infrastructure and the population of
childbearing women. These will range from countries such as
Bangladesh, where some 95% of the births are attended by
untrained traditional birth attendants or family members and
no civil registration exists (12), through countries like Niger,
with good primary health care records and poor civil
registration (13), Brazil with 75% coverage of civil
registration (14) and India, with a 1% sample registration
system (15, 16). Clearly no one method is the best in each of
these diverse situations. The choice of method will depend
not only on circumstances but also on the purposes for
which the data are to be used. Are they to be used for
monitoring over time? Or for planning health services and
infrastructure? Or for determining health care priorities? In
each case the degree of precision has to be balanced against
the cost in money and human resources.

It is possible to divide the methods into those that aim to
produce an estimate of the maternal mortality rate, for which
one needs an estimate of both the numerator (the number of
maternal deaths) and the denominator (the number of births),
which are here termed "direct" methods, and those that look
for a proxy measure which is indicative of the level of
maternal mortality—the "indirect" methods.

## Direct estimation methods

### Hospital data

The most commonly used alternative to using registration
data is to use hospital data to estimate the maternal
mortality rate in a larger catchment area. There are, however,
many limitations to this approach, and estimates calculated
on hospital data alone tend on the whole to be very high. In
general, the smaller the proportion of births taking place

inside the hospital the greater the discrepancy between the true—usually unknown—community rate and the hospital rate.

In Bogotá, Colombia, in 1971–73, deliveries at the Instituto Materno-Infantil accounted for 35% of all births in the city. The maternal mortality rate was 306 per 100 000 live births (17). During the same period the maternal mortality rate for the whole of Colombia was 190 per 100 000 (18). Bearing in mind that Bogotá probably has lower maternal mortality than the average for Colombia there remains a differential of about 2 to 1 in the two rates.

A similar example comes from Khartoum Province, Sudan, where in 1972 the overall rate for the Province was 320 per 100 000 live births, the institutional rate was 420 per 100 000 and the domiciliary rate was 300 per 100 000 (19). A few years later the rate at the Khartoum teaching hospital was 607 per 100 000, excluding deaths due to abortion (20).

The reason for such discrepancies between hospital and community mortality rates is that either the numerator (the women who died) or the denominator (the women who gave birth in the hospital) or both are not representative samples of all maternal deaths and of all women giving birth.

The usually upward bias found in rates coming from government (non-fee-paying) hospitals is due to two factors:

1. A large proportion of the women who die in such hospitals are emergency admissions, women who had intended to give birth at home but who were transported to hospital when they developed a life-threatening condition. Often they arrive too late and their deaths swell the number of hospital deaths. Women who gave birth safely at home do not of course appear in the denominator. This phenomenon emerges very clearly when hospital data are divided into booked and unbooked patients. At the Black Lion Hospital in Addis Ababa, Ethiopia, for example, the overall maternal mortality rate in 1980–81 was 960; for booked patients it was 210 compared with 1050 for unbooked patients.[1]

---

[1] Horvath, B. & Muletta, E. *Maternal mortality in Black Lion Hospital, 1981–1982.* Unpublished document of Department of Gynaecology and Obstetrics, Faculty of Medicine, Addis Ababa.

2. If a referral system is working efficiently, most high-risk women—at least those who present themselves for prenatal care—are referred to the hospital for delivery. This means that among the women giving birth at the hospital there is a disproportionate number of women with obstetric complications, and hence of women who die there. Those who have been referred to the hospital for delivery will appear in the statistics as booked patients. It is not possible, therefore, to estimate the degree of bias introduced into the maternal mortality rate as a result.

All this is not to suggest that hospital-based studies are of little value. On the contrary, valuable cause-of-death information can be obtained from this source which can shed some light at least on the need for specific interventions.

A third source of bias inherent in hospital rates is that of socioeconomic selection. If a hospital is fee-paying or caters for patients with a certain type of insurance, e.g., a private clinic or a military hospital, it will attract economically advantaged women. Such hospitals may have a lower maternal mortality rate than that prevailing in the community.

### Combining hospital data with data from other sources

The bias inherent in maternal mortality rates based on hospital data stems from the fact that the numerator and the denominator represent different population groups.

In places where the catchment area of the hospital is well defined and transport and cultural factors are such that most women in serious difficulty in childbirth, or following an abortion, are transported to hospital even if moribund, it is possible to assume that almost all maternal deaths take place in hospital. The number of such deaths can then be a good approximation to the numerator of the community maternal mortality rate. The problem of estimation then becomes one of defining the denominator, i.e., adding the estimated number of domiciliary births to the known number of hospital births. Rates derived in this fashion tend to be underestimates (because of the unknown number of deaths outside the hospital) but are very useful as minimum estimates. In Madras City, for example, during 1974 to 1975, there were some 393 maternal deaths and 87 438 deliveries in the four main teaching hospitals, giving a maternal mortality rate of 449 per 100 000. If instead of hospital deliveries the total number of births in the city—192 642—is used as denominator, the estimated maternal mortality rate for the city becomes 204 per 100 000 (*21*). This compares with the official estimate of 370 per 100 000 for the whole of India (*22*).

## Other health records

Numerous community studies testify to the fact that good records at the primary care level can provide all the information necessary for computing infant mortality rates for specific communities. Theoretically, maternal mortality rates can be calculated in the same way. The only difficulty is that of numbers. Even in countries with high maternal mortality rates a maternal death is a relatively rare event and to establish a maternal mortality rate of, for example, 300 per 100 000, correct to within 20% (95% confidence level), would require a sample size of 50 000 births.

The task is not impossible and several health development projects have produced reliable estimates of maternal mortality rates based on maternity records, but in most instances this has been as a by-product of other efforts. The keeping of records aimed only at measuring maternal mortality would place an unacceptable burden on already busy health workers and is not therefore a viable proposition.

Complete record coverage of all births is not very common in countries without registration systems. Nevertheless, a maternal death is a sufficiently memorable event for it to be possible to gather information on the number of maternal deaths occurring in a given area.

In a study in Bangladesh (*23*), specially trained interviewers visited health facilities (MCH centres, family planning clinics, hospitals, etc.) throughout Bangladesh to obtain reports about pregnancy-related deaths. Of the nearly 2000 reports only 40% were from hospitals. Family planning workers in rural clinics recalled more such deaths than did health workers in hospitals. Because family planning workers are most likely to know about reproductive health conditions they can be a very useful source of information. Even so, a comparison with the expected number of maternal deaths using a previous estimate of the maternal mortality rate for Bangladesh (*3*) showed considerable under-reporting of maternal deaths.

The earlier study mentioned above (3) had used matching of reports of adult female deaths, based on repeated household surveys, coupled with records of live births to estimate maternal mortality patterns and levels in a rural area of Bangladesh. Admittedly, this type of study is only possible for relatively small populations subject to intense field surveillance of vital events. None the less, inasmuch as the district (Matlab thana) was thought to be reasonably representative of health conditions throughout the country, this form of sample vital registration yielded extremely useful information and the resulting estimate of 570 maternal deaths per 100 000 live births remained the definitive estimate for Bangladesh until more recent community studies showed even this to be on the low side (24, 25).

In Niger the Ministry of Health has made an intensive effort to ensure that all deaths either occurring in health units or otherwise known to health personnel are registered, along with the cause of death. In addition, in 1980 all death records pertaining to deceased women of childbearing age were reviewed to ascertain whether maternal deaths were being correctly recorded. As a result, the coverage of maternal deaths was considered to be sufficiently accurate for a broad but none the less workable estimate of maternal mortality. Even in the absence of reasonably accurate records about the number of live births (civil registration of births is very incomplete), estimates of the denominator for calculating the maternal mortality rate can be derived, at least at a national level, from United Nations publications. Using a crude birth rate of 50 per 1000 as estimated for Niger to derive the expected annual number of live births led to an estimate of 135 maternal deaths per 100 000 live births, which was much more in accord with other estimates and was only about one-quarter of the rate (519 per 100 000) based on the number of recorded deliveries (13). The estimates derived in this way will be minimum rates: the degree of underestimation will depend on the completeness of the numerator.[1]

## Cause-of-death inquiries

A similar approach using field interviews was used to investigate causes of death among women of reproductive age in Egypt and Indonesia (4), India (26), Jamaica (27) and

---

[1] There has been some controversy as to the reasonableness of the Niger estimate, but this concerns the completeness of the numerator (29, 30).

Bangladesh (*24, 25*). These studies differ from that carried out earlier in Bangladesh (*3*) in one important aspect—non-medically trained people were used to interview the families of the deceased. In the Indonesian study, family planning field workers were trained to carry out the interviews. In the Egyptian study, where vital registration of the fact of death in the reproductive age group is likely to be reasonably good (*28*), deaths in women aged 15–50 years in the study area of Menoufia were first identified through the vital registration system. Interviews with the family of the deceased (most often the husband) were conducted on average between 30 and 40 days after death to ascertain the symptoms. The interview reports were then given to a panel of medical specialists for diagnosis. To estimate the maternal mortality rate in the district, the annual number of live births was derived by applying estimated age-specific fertility rates for Egypt as a whole to projections of the female population of Menoufia at these ages based on the latest available census results. The resulting estimate of maternal mortality was 263 per 100 000 live births, compared with the national rate of maternal mortality three years earlier, based on civil registration, of 79 per 100 000 (*5*). Looked at another way, the "official" rate was less than one-third of that found in Menoufia, a relatively privileged area of Egypt.

In Indonesia, family planning workers were asked to list all deaths in their villages during the previous month. This method proved less successful: only about half the estimated number of deaths were traced, those occurring in remote areas being under-represented (*10*). In the Bangladesh studies, which covered two rural areas, traditional midwives were asked to report all births and all deaths of women of reproductive age. These were followed up by supervisors who interviewed close relatives to ascertain the circumstances surrounding the death, including menstrual history preceding the death (to identify cases of early pregnancy and abortion) (*24, 25*).

In India and Jamaica, multiple sources of information were used to identify deaths of women of reproductive age (hospitals, civil registers, schools, mortuaries, etc.). Each death was then investigated to determine causes. A notable feature of these two studies was that no single source of information uncovered all the deaths.

All these inquiries used lay reporters and interviewers and a review panel which, after examining the lay reports regarding the symptoms leading to the death, assigned the cause of death to ICD categories. A similar procedure, but using health professionals as interviewers and tracing the deaths back through the health care system, was used some 20 years earlier to investigate the causes of adult mortality in 12 cities in the United Kingdom and North and South America (*31*). In every city it was found that maternal deaths had been underenumerated. Overall, some 30% of the final assignments to maternal causes had not originally been so classified. In eight cities the additions to maternal causes represented over a quarter of the final assignments.

## Household inquiries

Questions relating to maternal deaths can also be incorporated into one-off or repeated (large-scale) household inquiries. It is possible, for example, to ask questions on pregnancy status and to make a repeat visit one year later to ascertain the outcome of any pregnancy.

Alternatively, retrospective questions can be asked about household members. A recent community survey in Addis Ababa to identify births, abortions and deaths over a period of two years was based on a sample of households. These were then followed up and details of care received, social and other characteristics of the women and households, as well as circumstances and causes of deaths were recorded. A sample of nearly 10 000 pregnancies yielded 45 deaths and an estimated maternal mortality rate of 480 per 100 000. Nevertheless at the 95% level of significance this gives a sampling error of about 30%, i.e., the population rate could lie anywhere between 370 and 660 per 100 000 (*32, 33*).

Retrospective studies based on confidential questioning of husbands about the survival of their spouse have also been conducted. One such study of 30 000 husbands in Egypt, drawn from a rural area and the city of Alexandria, revealed that husbands could be a good source of information on maternal deaths.[1] The problem here, as elsewhere, is that those who are willing to collaborate in such an inquiry and who may be readily accessible are generally not representative of the population at large. Willingness to collaborate may also be very culture-specific. Moreover, there are a number

---

[1] El Sherbini, A. F. et al. *The feasibility of getting information about maternal mortality from the husband.* Unpublished document of the WHO Regional Office for the Eastern Mediterranean, 1983.

of theoretical questions to be overcome before such a method can be of practical use, in particular that of a denominator, which would require many more details of birth histories of all wives (surviving and deceased) than was collected in the pilot study. As with other studies the sample size required is very large.

## Indirect methods

There is considerable promise in the use of indirect methods to indicate high maternal mortality. Advances in demographic estimation techniques and improved health surveillance measures have yielded estimates of age- and sex-specific mortality rates for many countries, or areas within countries, where vital registration is poor or nonexistent. Higher mortality among women in the reproductive age group than among men of that age can, in the absence of knowledge about other factors, be taken as indicative of high maternal mortality. This does not, of course, yield a precise quantitative estimate of the level of maternal mortality but should be sufficient to indicate the order of magnitude of the problem.

The results of the record-matching study in Bangladesh vividly demonstrate the impact of maternity-related deaths on overall female mortality in the childbearing age group. Age-specific death rates derived for the study area are reproduced in Fig. 2.1. In the absence of maternity-related deaths, the age-specific death rates for the sexes would have been quite similar. However, when maternal deaths are included, overall death rates for females are roughly 50% higher at ages 20–34 years and 150% higher at ages 15–19 years (3).

While sex ratios of mortality (male death rate divided by the female death rate) markedly less than one are almost surely indicative of high maternal mortality, sex ratios close to one may well conceal a similar situation. Thus in societies where men are much more exposed to hazards at the workplace, accidental death rates for working-age men could be sufficiently high to counterbalance a high maternal mortality rate. Much the same effect could arise if male mortality from wars or other conflicts is particularly high.

Imbalanced population sex ratios can also be indicative of excess female mortality and, by implication, of high maternal mortality. Perhaps the best example of the use of this approach is a study of the census returns for India, Pakistan

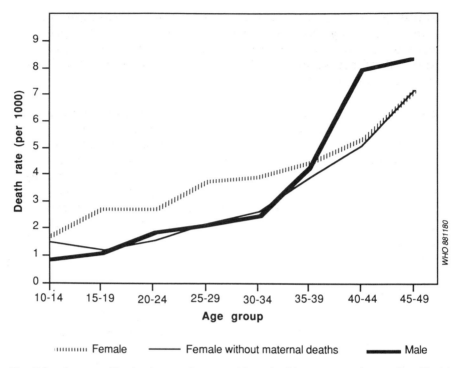

Fig. 2.1. Age-specific death rates by sex with and without maternal mortality, Matlab thana, Bangladesh, 1968–1970

and what was then Ceylon (*34*). Contrary to the normal pattern, population sex ratios (number of males divided by the number of females) *increased* with age in these countries so that at ages 45 years and over there were roughly 10–15% more men than women. At the childbearing ages (15–44 years), sex ratios were generally in the range 1.05–1.1.

Considerable caution is necessary in using this approach, however. In general it requires supportive evidence based on sex-specific mortality rates as well as information about sex differences in other confounding factors such as migration rates, under-reporting of births and deaths, and differential enumeration in the census.

Indirect estimates of male and female survival during adulthood can also be obtained using other demographic techniques. The United Nations has issued a convenient overview of these methods, including their data requirements and examples of their application (*35*). Essentially, these techniques permit the estimation of adult mortality based on information about either the orphanhood or widowhood status of respondents. Rather than providing estimates of conventional age-specific mortality rates, these techniques provide conditional probabilities of survival. The *relative survival* of the sexes can then be used to estimate the level of maternal mortality.

In addition to statistical techniques such as those described above, it is often possible to discover the frequency of maternal death using various social science techniques to elicit people's opinions on priority health problems.[1] Such techniques will not yield any quantitative estimates but may provide useful pointers. The clue may even lie in local folklore. As when Tanzanian mothers, about to give birth, bid their older children farewell, telling them "I am going to the sea to fetch a new baby, but the journey is long and dangerous and I may not return."

# References

1. MACFARLANE, A. & MUGFORD, M. *Birth counts: statistics of pregnancy and childbirth*, Vol. 1. London, Her Majesty's Stationery Office, 1984.

2. WORLD HEALTH ORGANIZATION. *International classification of diseases. Manual of the international statistical classification of diseases, injuries, and causes of death*. Ninth revision. Geneva, 1977.

3. CHEN, L. C. ET AL. Maternal mortality in rural Bangladesh. *Studies in family planning*, 5(11): 334–341 (1974).

4. FORTNEY, J. A. ET AL. *Causes of death to women of reproductive age in Egypt*. Michigan State University, 1984 (Working Paper No. 49).

5. UNITED NATIONS. *Demographic yearbook*. New York (various years).

6. ZISKIN, L. Z. ET AL. Improved surveillance of maternal deaths. *International journal of gynaecology and obstetrics*, 16: 282–286 (1979).

7. SMITH, J. C. ET AL. An assessment of the incidence of maternal mortality in the United States. *American journal of public health*, 74(8): 780–783 (1984).

8. RUBIN, G. ET AL. The risk of childbearing re-evaluated. *American journal of public health*, 71(7): 712–716 (1981).

9. SACHS, B. P. ET AL. Reproductive mortality in the United States. *Journal of the American Medical Association*, 247(20): 2789–2792 (1982).

---

[1] Coeytaux, F. *The role of the family in health: appropriate research methods.* Unpublished WHO document FHE/84.2.

10. FORTNEY, J. A. ET AL. Reproductive mortality in two developing countries. *American journal of public health*, **76**(2): 134–136 (1986).
11. WORLD HEALTH ORGANIZATION. *Lay reporting of health information*. Geneva, 1978.
12. BANGLADESH, MINISTRY OF HEALTH AND POPULATION CONTROL, MCH TASK FORCE. *National strategy for a comprehensive MCH programme*. Dhaka, 1985.
13. THURIAUX, M. C. & LAMOTTE, J.-M. Maternal mortality in developing countries: a note on the choice of denominator. *International journal of epidemiology*, **13**(2): 246–247 (1984).
14. BRAZIL, MINISTRY OF HEALTH, Secretaria Nacional de Ações Básicas de Saude, Divisão Nacional de Epidemiolgia. *Estatisticas de mortalidade, Brasil 1980*. Brasilia, Documentation Centre of the Ministry of Health, 1983.
15. INDIA, MINISTRY OF HOME AFFAIRS. *Vital statistics of India 1976* (16th issue). New Delhi, Office of Registrar General, 1981.
16. INDIA, MINISTRY OF HOME AFFAIRS. *Survey of causes of death (rural) 1979: a report* (Series 3, No. 12). New Delhi, Office of Registrar General, 1982.
17. SANCHEZ TORRES, F. Maternal mortality at the Mother and Child Institute, Bogotá (1971–1973). *Revista colombiana obstétrica y ginecológica*, **25**(6): 395–401 (1974).
18. PAN AMERICAN HEALTH ORGANIZATION. *Health conditions in the Americas, 1977–1980*. Washington, 1982 (PAHO Scientific Publication No. 427).
19. SUDAN, MINISTRY OF HEALTH. *Annual statistical report*, Khartoum, 1972.
20. ABBO, A. H. Preventable factors in maternal mortality in Khartoum Teaching Hospital. *Arab medical journal*, **4**(11, 12): 23–28 (1982).
21. BHASKER RAO, K. & MALIKA, P. E. A study of maternal mortality in Madras city. *Journal of obstetrics and gynaecology of India*, **27**(6): 876–880 (1977).
22. INDIA, MINISTRY OF HEALTH AND FAMILY WELFARE. *Family welfare programme in India: Yearbook 1979–1980*. New Delhi, 1981.
23. ROCHAT, R. W. ET AL. Maternal and abortion related deaths in Bangladesh, 1978–79. *International journal of gynaecology and obstetrics*, **19**: 155–164 (1981).
24. ALAUDDIN, M. Maternal mortality in rural Bangladesh. The Tangail District. *Studies in family planning*, **17**(1): 13–21 (1986).
25. KHAN, A. R. ET AL. Maternal mortality in rural Bangladesh. The Jamalpur district. *Studies in family planning*, **17**(1): 1–12 (1986).
26. BHATIA, J. C. *A study of maternal mortality in Anantapur district, Andhra Pradesh, India*. Bangalore, Indian Institute of Management, 1986.
27. WALKER, G. J. ET AL. Maternal mortality in Jamaica. *Lancet*, **1**(8479): 486–488 (1986).
28. NATIONAL RESEARCH COUNCIL. Committee on Population and

Demography. *The estimation of recent trends in fertility and mortality in Egypt.* Washington, National Academy Press, 1981 (Research report No. 9).

29. GRAY, R. H. Maternal mortality in developing countries (letter). *International journal of epidemiology,* **14**: 337 (1985).

30. JUNCKER, T. Maternal mortality in developing countries (letter). *International journal of epidemiology,* **14**: 338 (1985).

31. PUFFER, R. R. & WYNNE GRIFFITH, G. *Patterns of urban mortality.* Washington, DC, Pan American Health Organization, 1967 (PAHO Scientific Publication, No. 151).

32. KWAST, B. E. ET AL. Epidemiology of maternal mortality in Addis Ababa: a community-based study. *Ethiopian medical journal,* **23**(7): 7–16 (1985).

33. LWANGA, S. K. & LEMESHOW, S. *Sample size determination in health studies.* Geneva, World Health Organization, in press.

34. EL BADRY, M. A. Higher female than male mortality in some countries of south-east Asia: a digest. *American Statistical Association journal,* **64**(328): 1234–1244 (1969).

35. UNITED NATIONS POPULATION DIVISION & US NATIONAL ACADEMY OF SCIENCES. *Indirect techniques for demographic estimation.* New York, 1983 (ST/ESA/SER.A/81).

# Chapter 3

# THE DIMENSIONS OF THE PROBLEM

No one knows exactly how many women die each year as a result of becoming pregnant. Most of those who die are poor, they live in remote areas and their deaths are accorded little importance. In the parts of the world where maternal mortality is highest, deaths are rarely recorded and even if they are, the cause of death is usually not given.

Most of the evidence of high maternal mortality is fragmentary and indirect. Thus hospital data point to high rates but are misleading when it comes to exact levels. Civil registration data, where they exist, are almost always incomplete. It is now known, for example, that even in the USA, registration data underestimate the number of deaths by about 25% (1). Similarly, a recent independent study in Jamaica showed a rate more than twice as high as the official figure (2). For many countries there are national estimates of varying degrees of verisimilitude; some are "official" government or UN estimates, others just informed guesses. Fortunately, in recent years there have been a growing number of good community surveys which shed some light on the problem in places where very little was known before. In other areas a large number of orphaned children or many more female deaths than male deaths in the reproductive age groups may point to high levels of maternal mortality.

By approaching the information that is available in a pragmatic manner, it is possible to distinguish patterns and orders of magnitude which make up a formidable picture of the global dimensions of the problem (see Table 3.1). It is possible to estimate with a fair degree of certainty that each year at least half a million women die from causes related to pregnancy and childbirth. Over 99% of the maternal deaths—that is, all but about 6000—take place in developing countries, which account for 86% of the world's births. Well over half the maternal deaths occur in Asia, where nearly a third of a million women die each year. And three-quarters of these deaths occur in South Asia: in India, Pakistan and Bangladesh. There are, for example, more maternal deaths in

Table 3.1.   Estimated numbers of maternal deaths by region, about 1983

| Region | Estimated no. of deaths |
|---|---|
| *Developing countries* | |
| Africa | 150 000 |
| Northern Africa | 24 000 |
| Eastern Africa | 46 000 |
| Central Africa | 18 000 |
| Western Africa | 54 000 |
| Southern Africa | 8 000 |
| Asia | 308 000 |
| Southern Asia | 230 000 |
| Western Asia | 14 000 |
| Southeastern Asia | 52 000 |
| East Asia | 12 000 |
| Latin America | 34 000 |
| Central America | 9 000 |
| Caribbean | 2 000 |
| Tropical South America | 22 000 |
| Temperate South America | 1 000 |
| Oceania | 2 000 |
| Total | 494 000 |
| *Developed countries* | |
| Total | 6 000 |
| World total | 500 000 |

*Source*: Estimated numbers of births from United Nations (*9*).

India in one day than there are in all the developed countries in one month. Most of the remaining deaths—some 150 000 a year—occur in Africa.

# Africa

Maternal mortality rates, which measure the risk of dying from a given pregnancy, are highest in Africa, with community rates of up to 1000 per 100 000 live births reported in some rural areas. For example, a study carried out in four Gambian villages in 1982–83 found a rate in excess of 2000 per 100 000 (*3*). The Danfa project in Ghana estimated a maternal mortality rate of 400 per 100 000 in 1972 (*4*). And in a longitudinal study of a small rural area in Sine-Saloum, Senegal, in 1962–82 a rate of 700 per 100 000 was found (*5*).

The risk of dying from maternal causes is somewhat lower in the urban areas of Africa, though rates of over 500 per

100 000 live births have been reported in several cities. A recent study in Addis Ababa, for example, revealed a rate of 566 per 100 000 (6), and Accra is estimated to have had a rate of 800 per 100 000 in 1974 (7).

National estimates vary between about 1100 per 100 000 (in Somalia)[1] and 52 per 100 000 (in Mauritius) (8). In general, maternal mortality rates in Northern and Southern Africa are a little lower than in Western, Central and Eastern Africa. This is very much in line with what is known of women's life expectancy and overall death rates. Basing estimates on these and extrapolating for areas for which we do not yet have community data, the best estimates for the number of deaths per 100 000 live births in each of the subregions of Africa are:

| | |
|---|---|
| Northern Africa | 500 |
| Western Africa | 700 |
| Eastern Africa | 660 |
| Central Africa | 690 |
| Southern Africa | 570 |
| Overall | 640 |

In Africa high maternal mortality rates are compounded by high fertility. The average number of live births per woman is 6.4 (9). But in rural Africa it is quite common for a woman to have given birth to eight live babies and to have been pregnant several more times. If, at each pregnancy, such a woman has a one in 140 chance of dying (calculated for a maternal mortality rate of 700 per 100 000), she has a lifetime risk of dying from pregnancy-related causes of at least one in 15.

## Asia

Very high rates of maternal mortality are also found in Southern Asia. Two recent community studies in rural Bangladesh—in Jamalpur (10) and in the Tangail District (11)—found rates of approximately 623 and 566 per 100 000 live births, respectively. The Government of Pakistan estimated the national rate to lie between 600 and 800 per 100 000 in 1978 (12). A 1984–85 study in Andhra Pradesh, India, found a rate of 874 per 100 000 in rural areas and 545 per 100 000 in urban areas (13). Extremely high rates have

---

[1] *Report on expanded programme on immunization and maternal and child health in Somali Democratic Republic.* Unpublished WHO document EM/IMZ/20, EM/MCH/159, EM/SOM/EPI/001.

also been reported from remote areas of Nepal (*14*).[1] The
exception in this region is Sri Lanka with a maternal
mortality rate of 95 per 100 000 in 1980 (WHO data). With a
high population density and high maternal mortality rates,
South Asia accounts for 41% of the world's births and 59%
of its maternal deaths, even though fertility rates in the
region are not quite as high as in Africa. The average
woman in all countries of this area except Sri Lanka can
expect to have over 6 live births and perhaps 8 or 9
pregnancies during her lifetime. Her lifetime chance of dying
from pregnancy-related causes is about one in 18.

In contrast, maternal mortality rates in East Asia are quite
low, with China reporting a rate of 59 per 100 000 in rural
areas and 25 per 100 000 in urban areas of 21 provinces (*15*).
Hong Kong and Singapore have rates in line with the lowest
in Europe (6 per 100 000 and 11 per 100 000, respectively).
The rate in Japan has halved in the last ten years and is
now about 15 per 100 000 (*16*).

Rates in Southeastern and Western Asia, while on average
not as high as in Southern Asia, are still in excess of 700
per 100 000 in some areas. In Bali, for instance, a recent
study found a rate of 718 per 100 000 (*17*). Rates are also
high in Democratic Yemen, where the government estimate is
1000 per 100 000, and in the Syrian Arab Republic, where
the UNFPA estimate is 280 per 100 000 (*18*), though the
registration data give a rate of 7 per 100 000 (*19*). In the
Philippines, civil registration data gave a rate of 80 per
100 000 in 1984 (WHO data), but this is also likely to be an
underestimate. UNICEF estimates a rate of 110 per 100 000
for Viet Nam (*20*), but a 1972 study found a rate of 378 per
100 000 in Saigon (*21*). Government data for Peninsular
Malaysia gave a rate of 63 per 100 000 in 1980 (*22*), and a
rate of 14 per 100 000 has been reported for Kuala Lumpur.[2]
Both estimates exclude abortion-related deaths. Rates in the
oil-producing countries have dropped to quite low levels, such
as 18 per 100 000 in Kuwait and 19 per 100 000 in Bahrain
(*16, 23*).

Asia is thus the continent with the greatest contrasts.
Differences found here are as great as those between the

---

[1] Wright, N. *Epidemiologic review of data on primary health problems in Nepal:
report.* Unpublished document, 1986.
[2] Adeeb, N. *Report on maternal mortality for Selangor and Kuala Lumpur in 1982
and 1983.* Unpublished document of the National University of Malaysia, 1984.

richest and the poorest countries of the whole world. The best estimates for the average numbers of maternal deaths per 100 000 live births in each of the subregions are:

| | |
|---|---|
| Western Asia | 340 |
| Southern Asia | 650 |
| Southeastern Asia | 420 |
| East Asia | 55 |
| Overall | 420 |

Among the countries with very high mortality rates there are some where, because fertility is moderate, a woman will be at less risk over her lifetime of dying from pregnancy-related causes than a woman in a country where both maternal mortality and fertility rates are high. Thus in Bali, where the maternal mortality rate is over 700 per 100 000, a woman has a lifetime risk of dying from pregnancy-related causes of one in 32, while a woman in Bangladesh, with a maternal mortality rate of 600 but a much higher average number of live births, has a one in 26 chance of dying as a result of pregnancy.

## Latin America

Most of the data for Latin America are based on civil registration and therefore tend to be underestimates. An Inter-American Investigation of Mortality carried out some twenty years ago showed that in the Latin American cities investigated, maternal deaths were often reported as being due to other causes (24). This was particularly true of abortion-related deaths. In Bogotá, for instance, the official rate for abortion-related deaths was 79 per 100 000 live births, whereas the investigators found a rate of 126 per 100 000. A particularly striking feature of this study was indeed the high proportion of maternal deaths that were due to abortion, ranging from 13% in Lima, Peru, to 53% in Santiago, Chile.

The highest rates based on vital registration are to be found in Ecuador (220 per 100 000) (25) and Paraguay (469 per 100 000) (26). A high rate has also been reported by Government sources in Peru (27), where it was 314 per 100 000 in 1984. In Haiti, a Government project found a rate of 367 per 100 000 in 1974–78 (28). However, a recent community survey in Jamaica (2) found a rate of 102 per 100 000, which was double the official figure. Rates can also vary considerably within a country. Thus in Manaus, north-east Brazil, a rate of 310 per 100 000 is reported, compared with 99 per 100 000 in rural São Paulo State (29).

As elsewhere, maternal mortality in Latin America is in line with the general patterns of mortality, aggravated perhaps by high levels of abortion in many places. Overall, the lowest levels are to be found in temperate areas, and the highest in tropical South America. The regional estimates are as follows:

| | |
|---|---|
| Central America | 240 |
| Caribbean | 220 |
| Tropical South America | 310 |
| Temperate South America | 110 |
| Overall | 270 |

## Developed countries

Maternal mortality rates in western and northern Europe, based on civil registration data, are mostly about 10 per 100 000 or lower—the lowest in the world. Iceland and Luxembourg actually had no maternal deaths in the latest year for which data are available. Rates in southern and eastern Europe are slightly higher but, with the notable exception of Romania, which has a very high rate of mortality due to abortion, they are only rarely more than 30 per 100 000. Rates in Australia, Canada, Japan, New Zealand and the USA are in line with those in Europe. The USSR has a rate of 48 per 100 000 (WHO data). Allowing for under-registration, for which there is now ample evidence, it is estimated that the developed countries as a whole have a maternal mortality rate of about 30 per 100 000 live births. Coupled with low fertility this means that, at most, 6000 maternal deaths a year—or just over 1% of the total—occur in the developed world.

## Historical evidence of high rates

Some of the extremely high rates quoted by researchers in developing countries beg the question of what proportion of women would die in childbirth, or from pregnancy-related causes generally, if there were no health care and if their general health status were poor. Rates of over 1000 per 100 000 have been quoted in many remote areas: 1000 in Tunisia (30), 2000 in Gambia (3), 1400 in Ghana (31), 1500 in Nigeria (official data), 2000 in Nepal (14) and 1360 in

India.[1] Are these possible, or are they just wild guesses? A comparison with rates pertaining many years ago in the developed countries indicates that the figures may be quite realistic. For example, in eighteenth century rural France the maternal mortality rate was well over 1000 per 100 000 (*32*), as was also the case in Sweden (*33*). A study of the ruling families of Europe showed a rate of about 2000 per 100 000 between the years 1500 and 1850 (*32*).

A careful analysis of the records from three rural churches in England dating from the 16th to the 18th century produced an estimated rate of 27 maternal deaths per 1000 baptisms— which also indicates a maternal mortality rate of over 2000 per 100 000 births (*34*). The earliest data published by the Registrar-General for England and Wales refer to the year 1840. From then till the end of the century the (registered) maternal mortality rate varied between 400 and 600 per 100 000. The rates in some counties, however, were considerably higher, reaching 900 per 100 000 in remoter areas. Again, all these statistics are likely to be underestimates. Until 1935 the rate for England and Wales (based on vital registration) remained fairly constant at about 400 per 100 000 (*35*).

In the light of these figures, the very high rates reported from remote areas today appear quite plausible. With no knowledge of asepsis, no means of dealing with life-threatening complications (no caesarean sections, no blood transfusions, no antibiotics), poor nutrition, hard physical work, large families and closely spaced pregnancies, rates are bound to be high. Some workers in the field have gone as far as to define a "physiological norm" of approximately 1200 maternal deaths per 100 000 live births against which to measure risk reduction.

## The contribution of maternal mortality to overall mortality

In most developing countries, between a quarter and a third of the deaths of women in their reproductive years can be attributed to maternal causes. But the proportion can be even higher. In some rural areas of South Asia, of every two women that die one will have died because she became

---

[1] *Bulletin of regional health information.* Unpublished WHO document SEA/VHS/165 Rev. 1.

pregnant. These proportions are all the more striking when one remembers that in such areas overall mortality—from infectious diseases, accidents, etc.—is already very high. Death is a very common event, and for women living in the poorer parts of the world, maternal mortality augments the risk of dying by at least one-third, and in some remote rural areas by as much as 85%. Such high risks associated with childbearing affect female life expectancy, and it is only when the latter reaches 55 or 60 years that maternal mortality can be assumed to be making less contribution to overall mortality (see Table 3.2).

Table 3.2. Maternal deaths as a proportion of all deaths of women of reproductive age

| Area | Deaths from pregnancy-related causes (%)[a] | Maternal mortality rate (per 100 000 live births) | Year | Source |
|---|---|---|---|---|
| Bangladesh, rural Jamalpur | 46 | 623 | 1982–3 | 10 |
| India, rural Andhra Pradesh | 45 | 874 | 1984–5 | 13 |
| Bangladesh, rural Tangail | 33 | 566 | 1982–3 | 11 |
| India, urban Andhra Pradesh | 28 | 545 | 1984–5 | 13 |
| Paraguay | 27 | 275 | 1984 | 19 |
| Bangladesh, Matlab | 26 | 510 | 1983 | b |
| Indonesia, Bali | 23 | 718 | 1980–2 | 17 |
| Egypt, Menoufia | 23 | 190 | 1981–3 | 17 |
| Egypt, South | 21 | 300 | 1984–5 | c |
| Ecuador | 16 | 190 | 1980 | 19 |
| Romania | 10 | 149 | 1984 | 19 |
| Mexico | 10 | 88 | 1984 | 19 |
| El Salvador | 8 | 70 | 1984 | 19 |
| Mauritius | 6 | 103 | 1985 | 19 |
| Costa Rica | 5 | 26 | 1983 | 19 |
| Cuba | 3 | 45 | 1983 | 19 |
| Japan | 1 | 16 | 1985 | 19 |
| USA | 1 | 8 | 1903 | 19 |
| Hong Kong | 1 | 5 | 1985 | 19 |
| Sweden | 0 | 2 | 1984 | 19 |

[a] Relative to all deaths among women of reproductive age.
[b] Lindpainter, L. S. et al. *Maternal mortality in Matlab Thana, Bangladesh, 1982.* Unpublished document of the International Centre for Diarrhoeal Diseases Research, Dhaka, Bangladesh.
[c] Abdullah, S. A. et al. Maternal mortality in upper Egypt. In: *Interregional Meeting on the Prevention of Maternal Mortality, Geneva 11–15 November 1985.* Unpublished WHO document FHE/PMM/85.9.18

## High-risk women

Even within a given social setting not all pregnant women run an equal risk; some are more likely to die than others. Everywhere in the world various behavioural and biological factors increase the risk of a woman developing life-threatening complications. Apart from such significant factors as a woman's stature and her nutritional and health status, the most easily recognized and the most universally significant factors are the woman's age and the number of her previous pregnancies. Despite the fact that in the more privileged countries of the world most obstetric complications are satisfactorily treated, the additional risk associated with these factors persists. The magnitude of the added risk may, however, vary between population groups.

Extreme youth significantly increases the risk of childbearing the world over. World Fertility Survey reports show that teenage marriage is widespread in the developing world, with the highest recorded incidence in Bangladesh, where 90% of women are married before they are 18 years old. Half of the women born in the late 1950s were in fact married before they were 15 years old. By the age of 17, almost half of all women in Bangladesh are mothers, and by the age of 19, one-third have at least two children. A survey carried out in Matlab, Bangladesh showed that girls aged 10–14 years had a maternal mortality rate five times higher than women aged 20 to 24, and that for those aged 15–19 the rate was twice as high as for 20–24-year-olds (*36*). During 1968–70 over half the observed mortality in women aged 15–19 in Bangladesh was due to maternal causes. Similar patterns exist in Africa. In Zaria, Nigeria, the under-15s had a maternal mortality nearly 7 times that of women aged 20 to 24, while for 16-year-olds it was 2.5 times higher (*37*). Even in the USA, girls under 15 have a maternal mortality rate three times that of women aged 20–24 years (*38*).

At the other end of the scale, the risk associated with childbearing begins to rise again after the age of 30 or 35. In a study in the USA women aged 40 to 44 had a maternal mortality nearly ten times higher than women aged 24 and 25 (*38*). In Matlab, Bangladesh, women aged over 40 years ran twice the risk of women aged 20–24 years (*36*), while in Zaria the risk for women aged 30 was already two-and-a-half times that for women of 20 to 24 (*37*). The excess risk to older women is particularly significant because in many parts of the world births to women aged over 35 make up a sizeable proportion of all births; the figures are 15% in Nigeria, 17% in Senegal, 25% in Bangladesh, 11% in Sri Lanka and 21% in the USA (16).

Whatever the age of the mother, second and third births are the safest, while the risks increase with subsequent pregnancies. In Matlab, the sixth and subsequent births were found to have an associated maternal mortality rate three times that of second births. In Jamaica the maternal mortality rate for sixth and subsequent births was twice that of second births. Unlike risky first births, which can only be accorded greater care but cannot be avoided, many high-parity births are unplanned and may be unwanted. Family planning therefore has its greatest scope for reducing the risk associated with childbearing at this end of the spectrum.

## The role of fertility

A large proportion of the half million maternal deaths take place each year because women are having more pregnancies than they want. The World Fertility Survey, carried out in the late 1970s in 40 developing countries, asked women whether they wanted any more children. If all those who said they wanted no more were actually able to stop childbearing, the number of births would be reduced by about 35% in Latin America, 33% in Asia and 17% in Africa.[1] At the very least, the number of maternal deaths would fall by an equivalent amount, but more likely it would fall even further, for three reasons. First and most importantly, there would be very few deaths due to induced abortion. Many studies have shown that abortion-related deaths account for a very large proportion of maternal mortality: over half in some Latin American cities, over a quarter in Addis Ababa (6), and a fifth in rural Bangladesh (10), for example. Secondly, the very fact that a pregnancy is unwanted carries an added risk. Women with unwanted pregnancies are less likely than other women to seek prenatal care or to deliver with a trained attendant. Lastly, women who want no more children tend to be older and have a higher parity, which means that they have a higher than average risk of maternal mortality. All in all, it would seem that if women were able to avoid

---

[1] Maine, D. et al. *Prevention of maternal deaths in developing countries: program options and practical considerations.* Paper prepared for the International Safe Motherhood Conference, Nairobi, 10–13 February 1987.

unwanted pregnancy, at the very least a quarter of the maternal deaths that occur each year would be avoided: each year some 150 000 women would not die.

## Trends in maternal mortality rates

It is very difficult to paint a global picture of trends in maternal mortality. Vital registration data exist in only 69 of the 166 Member States of WHO, covering less than one-third of the world's population. For the remaining countries there are rarely comparable studies that allow valid comparisons over time. Nevertheless, a few general trends are discernible. It is possible to see, for example, that maternal mortality rates have declined significantly in almost all developed countries in recent years. Table 3.3 shows such trends for a selection of countries.

Table 3.3.  Trends in maternal mortality rates, selected countries

| Country | Maternal mortality per 100 000 live births (MMR) | | Change | Latest available MMR |
|---|---|---|---|---|
| | 1965 | 1975 | | |
| Czechoslovakia | 35 | 18 | −49% | 8 (1982) |
| France | 23 | 20 | −13% | 13 (1980) |
| Federal Republic of Germany | 69 | 40 | −42% | 11 (1983) |
| Greece | 46 | 19 | −59% | 12 (1982) |
| Japan | 88 | 29 | −67% | 15 (1983) |
| Portugal | 85 | 43 | −48% | 15 (1984) |
| Romania | 86 | 121 | +41% | 149 (1984) |
| Romania (excluding abortion) | 65 | 31 | −52% | 21 (1984) |
| USA | 32 | 13 | −59% | 9 (1980) |

*Source*: World Health Organization: data reported by Member States.

The Ten-Year Health Plan for the Americas set a target for the reduction of maternal mortality rates by 1980. An appraisal of the results shows that, while rates declined in all countries over the period 1970–80, the greatest reductions were achieved in Costa Rica, Chile, Puerto Rico, Nicaragua and Honduras (*39*).

In Asia there are very few countries with reliable data. Maternal mortality rates have declined considerably in Hong Kong and Singapore, both of which now have rates in line with developed countries. Sri Lanka is an interesting success story. From a level of 555 per 100 000 in 1950–55, the maternal mortality rate fell to 239 per 100 000 ten years later and to 95 per 100 000 in 1980. In 1950–55 one-quarter of maternal deaths (other than those due to abortion) were due to sepsis, a ratio that is not uncommon in situations of high mortality. By 1977 the proportion had fallen to 10%.

Unlike the rapid decline in deaths from sepsis, deaths from haemorrhage declined more slowly, particularly in the early years, which indicates that haemorrhage as a cause of maternal mortality is less easy to prevent. No doubt the fact that 85% of births in Sri Lanka are now attended by trained people, and 76% take place in institutions[1] provides at least part of the explanation for the fall in maternal mortality.

There is little evidence of any decline in Africa. In some areas rates found in community studies have turned out to be lower than was assumed to be the case—in rural Senegal, for instance, a community study by ORSTOM (unpublished data, 1986) gave a figure of 590 per 100 000, whereas a rate of 700 had previously been reported (5). In other areas, rates have turned out to be higher than expected.

In sum, it would appear that while countries that currently have rates below, say, 100 per 100 000 have experienced recent falls in the maternal mortality rate, there is very little evidence of progress in countries with a higher mortality.

## The challenge

The high maternal mortality in poor countries relative to that in rich ones is a result of two factors— high fertility and a high risk of dying each time a woman becomes pregnant. The two tend to go together, although not always. It is useful to keep the two concepts separate because, while each has its roots in poverty, they require quite distinct action to combat them.

The risk of dying as a result of a given pregnancy in the richest developed countries is at least 100 times lower than in the poorest countries of Africa and Asia. If women the world over had the same chances of survival when they became pregnant as do women in the developed world, 460 000 fewer women would die, 1.5 million children would not lose their mothers, and undoubtedly millions more women would be

---

[1] *Report of the EMR/SEAR meeting on prevention of neonatal tetanus.* Unpublished WHO document EM/IMZ/27, EM/BD/14, EM-SEA/MTG.PREV.NNL.TTN./81.

spared lifelong handicaps. If, on the other hand, nothing is done to make childbearing safer, to decrease the number of unwanted pregnancies, or the dangers of illegal abortion, the number of women dying from pregnancy-related causes will increase with the number of women in the reproductive age group: in 1999 nearly 600 000 women will die, and between 1987 and the end of the century maternal mortality will claim another 7.5 million women.

# References

1. ZISKIN, L. Z. ET AL. Improved surveillance of maternal deaths. *International journal of gynaecology and obstetrics*, **16**: 282–286 (1979).

2. WALKER, G. J. ET AL. Maternal mortality in Jamaica. *Lancet*, **1** (8479): 486–488 (1986).

3. GREENWOOD, A. ET AL. A prospective study of pregnancy in a rural area of the Gambia, West Africa. *Bulletin of the World Health Organization*, **65**(5): 635–644 (1987).

4. AMPOFO, D. A. ET AL. The training of traditional birth attendants in Ghana: experience of the Danfa rural health project. *Tropical and geographical medicine*, **29**(2): 197–203 (1977).

5. FAMILY HEALTH INTERNATIONAL. Study of maternal mortality in Senegal. *Network*, **5**(1): 2 (1983).

6. KWAST, B. E. ET AL. Epidemiology of maternal mortality in Addis Ababa: a community-based study. *Ethiopian medical journal*, **23**(7): 7–16 (1985).

7. OJO, O. A. & SAVAGE, V. Y. A ten-year review of maternal mortality rates in the University Hospital, Ibadan, Nigeria. *American journal of obstetrics and gynecology*, **118**(4): 517–522 (1974).

8. MAURITIUS, MINISTRY OF HEALTH. *Vital and health statistics of the island of Mauritius: 1980*. Port Louis, 1981.

9. UNITED NATIONS. *Demographic indicators of countries: estimates and projections as assessed in 1980*. New York, Department of International Economic and Social Affairs, 1982.

10. KHAN, A. R. ET AL. Maternal mortality in rural Bangladesh. *World health forum*, **6**: 325–328 (1985).

11. ALAUDDIN, M. Maternal mortality in rural Bangladesh. The Tangail District. *Studies in family planning*, **17**(1): 13–21 (1986).

12. PAKISTAN, PLANNING COMMISSION, PLANNING AND DEVELOPMENT DIVISION. *Health and health-related statistics of Pakistan*. 2nd ed. Islamabad, Printing Corporation of Pakistan Press, 1978.

13. BHATIA, J. C. *A study of maternal mortality in Anantapur district, Andhra Pradesh, India*. Bangalore, Indian Institute of Management, 1986.

14. SHAH, M. *Rural health needs: report of a study in the primary health care unit (district) of Dhankuta, Nepal*. Kathmandu, Tribhuvan University, 1977.

15. ZHANG, L. & DING, H. China: analysis of cause and rate of regional maternal death in 21 provinces, municipalities and autonomous regions. *Chinese journal of obstetrics and gynaecology*, **21**(4): 195–197 (1986).

16. UNITED NATIONS. *Demographic yearbook*. New York (various years).

17. FORTNEY, J. A. ET AL. Reproductive mortality in two developing countries. *American journal of public health*, **76**(2): 134–136 (1986).

18. UNITED NATIONS FUND FOR POPULATION ACTIVITIES. *Syrian Arab Republic: report of second mission on needs assessment for population assistance*. New York, 1985.

19. *World health statistics annual, 1986*. Geneva, World Health Organization, 1986.

20. UNITED NATIONS ECONOMIC AND SOCIAL COMMISSION FOR ASIA AND THE PACIFIC. *The Asian and Pacific atlas of children in national development, 1984*. Bangkok, United Nations Children's Fund, 1984.

21. FROMENTIN, J. *South Vietnam: health*. Paris, Centre International de l'Enfance, 1974.

22. MALAYSIA, DEPARTMENT OF STATISTICS. *Monthly statistical bulletin, September 1982*. Kuala Lumpur, 1982.

23. BAHRAIN, MINISTRY OF HEALTH. *Annual report 1981*. Bahrain, 1982.

24. PUFFER, R. R. & WYNNE GRIFFITH, G. *Patterns of urban mortality*, Washington, DC, 1967 (PAHO Scientific Publication No. 151).

25. ECUADOR, INSTITUTO NACIONAL DE ESTADÍSTICA Y CENSOS. *Encuesta anual de estadísticas vitales· nacimientos y defunciones, 1978*. Quito, 1981.

26. PAN AMERICAN HEALTH ORGANIZATION. *Health conditions in the Americas, 1977–1980*. Washington, DC, 1982 (PAHO Scientific Publication No. 427).

27. JIMENEZ LA ROSA, R. E. *Participación de la mujer peruana en la salud y el desarrollo*. Lima, Ministry of Health, 1984.

28. BERGGREN, G. G. ET AL. Traditional midwives, tetanus immunization and infant mortality in rural Haiti. *Tropical doctor*, **13**(2): 79–87 (1983).

29. LACRETA, O. & MARETTI, M. Mortalidade materna. *Revista brasileira de medicina*, **39**(3): 89–106 (1982).

30. UNITED NATIONS FUND FOR POPULATION ACTIVITIES. *Report of mission on needs assessment for population assistance—Tunisia*. New York, 1981.

31. GHANA, MINISTRY OF HEALTH. *A primary health care strategy for Ghana*. Accra, National Health Planning Unit, 1978.

32. GUTIERREZ, H. & HOUDAILLE, J. La mortalité maternelle en France au XVIIIe siècle. *Population*, **6**: 975–994 (1983).

33. HOGBERG, U. *Maternal mortality in Sweden*. Umea, Sweden, Umea University, 1985.

34. DOBBIE, B. M. An attempt to estimate the true rate of maternal

mortality, sixteenth to eighteenth centuries. *Medical history*, **26**: 79–90 (1982).

35. MACFARLANE A. & MUGFORD, M. *Birth counts: statistics of pregnancy and childbirth.* Vol. 1. London, Her Majesty's Stationery Office, 1984.

36. CHEN, L. C. ET AL. Maternal mortality in rural Bangladesh. *Studies in family planning*, **5**(11): 334–341 (1974).

37. HARRISON, K. A. Childbearing, health and social priorities. A survey of 22,774 consecutive births in Zaria, Northern Nigeria. *British journal of obstetrics and gynaecology*, Supplement No. 5 (1985).

38. ROCHAT, R. W. Maternal mortality in the United States of America. *World health statistics quarterly*, **34**: 2–13 (1981).

39. PAN AMERICAN HEALTH ORGANIZATION. *Health of women in the Americas.* Washington, DC, 1985 (PAHO Scientific Publication, No. 488).

# Chapter 4

# THE STATUS OF WOMEN AND MATERNAL MORTALITY

A woman's status and her health are intricately entwined. Any serious attempt to improve the health of women—if it is to succeed—must deal firstly with those ways in which a woman's health is harmed by social customs and cultural traditions simply because she was born female (1).

Somewhere in the developing world a woman dies in childbirth and the cause of death entered on her medical record card is haemorrhage, or eclampsia, or perhaps sepsis. Such a record gives the impression that the woman's death was a tragic misfortune, a chance event unrelated to anything but the risky process of childbirth itself. This is a false impression. Maternal mortality should not be viewed as a chance event so much as a chronic disease developing over a long period, for the outcome of a pregnancy is profoundly influenced by the circumstances of a woman's life, by the economic and environmental conditions in which she lives, as well as by her social status.

The "status of women" is hard to pin down as a concept because it includes both practical and psychological aspects and involves a complex set of inter-related factors. A woman's status is often described in terms of her income, employment, education, health and fertility, as well as the roles she plays within the family, the community and society. It also involves society's perception of these roles and the value it places upon them. The status of women implies a comparison with the status of men and is therefore a significant reflection of the level of social justice in a society. This concept of social justice inherent in the term "status of women" is particularly important to the present analysis.

Typically, where rates of maternal death are high the social status of women is low; their needs have been ignored altogether or have taken second place to those of men since childhood. The link is not coincidental, yet sex discrimination as a contributory factor to maternal mortality has been largely ignored. It has been hidden within the general issue of poverty and underdevelopment which is assumed to put everyone—men, women, and children—at an equal disadvantage in health terms. The fact that the richest sources of information about maternal mortality are the hospitals means that the focus of attention has been on its biomedical and clinical causes rather than on its sociocultural context.

The UN Decade for Women (1976–85) did much to open the eyes of the world to the effects of sex discrimination on such things as economic development and the health of families, and many useful insights can be gained from the information that has begun to appear. But there is now a pressing need to establish the relationship between the status of women and maternal mortality.

The stereotype of the woman with low status is the woman with a child at the breast, another on the way and several more children playing round her skirts. It is the woman for whom marriage and motherhood have been her only destiny from birth; not to have achieved them would have carried an unbearable stigma. It is the woman who looks old beyond her years, and who is in poor health from the constant demands of pregnancy, motherhood and domestic work. Very probably she will be responsible for growing the family's food as well as preparing it, or working for wages outside the home just to make ends meet. Typically, too, such a woman will have very little, if any, education, and neither title to, nor prospect of inheriting, the family land on which she works, or the house in which she lives.

This picture is like a tapestry made up of millions of threads so intricately woven that cause and effect are extremely hard to trace. However, it is possible to draw out several major threads, and to see what contribution they make to maternal mortality. They could be called the causes behind the causes, and they involve unregulated fertility, educational status, and factors that affect the general health of women.

## Too many children, too early, too late and too close together

In Kenya the average number of babies born to each woman is eight. This is the highest fertility rate in the world: the average for Africa as a whole is 6.5, Asia 4.1 and Latin America 4.3, compared with 1.9 for the developed countries

(2). However, averages mask huge variations and it is not uncommon to meet women in the villages of India, Brazil or Burkina Faso who have borne ten or more children.

Contrary to the popular belief that childbirth gets easier with each experience of it, the risks involved in repeated childbearing are many. The second and third births are the most trouble-free, while the risk of serious complications, such as haemorrhage, rupture of the uterus and infection, rises steadily from the third birth onwards.

The years 20–30 are the safest period of a woman's life for childbearing, though between 10% and 20% of babies born in developing countries are to women in their teens who may be little more than children themselves. One study found, for example, that even two years after the onset of menstruation a girl may have between 2% and 9% of pelvic growth and 1% of height still to achieve (3). Not surprisingly, obstructed delivery due to disproportion between the size of the infant's head and the mother's pelvis (cephalopelvic disproportion) is most common among these very young mothers.

Because their bodies are not yet fully prepared for the demands of childbirth, teenagers run an excess risk of death compared with women aged 20–24 years. In a study in Nigeria, for example, women aged 15 had a maternal mortality rate 7 times that of women aged 20–24(4). Childbearing is more hazardous for older women also. For example, the risk of death in Jamaica was doubled for women of 30–34 years and increased five-fold for women over 40 years compared with women aged 20–24 years (5). Of course, the degree of risk to any one woman is enormously affected by her socioeconomic circumstances—her general state of health as well as her access to good quality professional health care. Thus, a 42-year-old Swedish woman faces a far less hazardous prospect in giving birth than, say, a 20-year-old woman in a remote village in Nigeria.

Where socioeconomic conditions are poor, women are most vulnerable to the health risks associated with bearing children in quick succession. Pregnancy and breast-feeding make big nutritional demands that women from poor homes are seldom able to meet either by eating more or by getting more rest.

It is estimated that a woman already in good health and. only moderately active requires about 300 extra calories a day during pregnancy, if she has not modified her energy output, as well as an increased supply of vitamins, folic acid, iron and other minerals. For the first six months of breast-feeding the extra calorie requirement is approximately 550 per day for a woman who was well nourished during pregnancy and who has thus been able to lay down reserves, particularly during the last three months (6).

For millions of women in developing countries, however, these figures are purely academic. The reality is that they never get enough food or rest for good health, and pregnancy and breast-feeding take a big toll on their bodies. Lack of time to recuperate between pregnancies compounds the problem. Thin, apathetic women with lustreless hair and skin, and sores that are slow to heal are not uncommon among those with large families in poor areas of the developing world. Many studies describe them, and in Bangladesh there is even a special name for such a condition. Commonly these women lack both protein and energy, and are also anaemic.

Women in their reproductive years require three times as much iron per day as do adult men. However, few get as much as they need and in poor communities the prevalence of infection and parasitic diseases compounds the problem. It is estimated that while half the non-pregnant women of the developing world are clinically anaemic, two-thirds of those who are pregnant suffer from the condition (7). Because it starves the body of oxygen, anaemia makes women tired and listless, but it also increases the danger from haemorrhage and other complications in childbirth.

It is particularly important for the survival chances of the fetus that the mother rests and gains weight during the last three months of pregnancy. However, a study of 202 widely different societies revealed that, in most, women continued their full work and activities right up to birth, and generally resumed them a very short time after giving birth (8). In the Gambia, where women are responsible for all the manual labour in the rice fields, they have been found actually to lose weight during the last three months of pregnancy if it happens to coincide with the busiest time in the fields (9). In fact, most studies bear witness to the fact that the women in poorest physical shape and therefore in most need of rest during pregnancy are least likely to get it.

The important question as far as the social causes of maternal death are concerned is *why* women bear many children and fail to have a reasonable recuperative period between pregnancies. One answer is that in spite of the costs to their health, many women believe it to be in their own best interests, for a variety of reasons.

## Children that prove a woman's worth

In many patriarchal societies a woman's only path to social status and personal achievement is through motherhood. Where this is held to be the only proper role for women, all the social mechanisms will operate on that principle, cutting off other options for girls from birth. There will be little commitment to their education, and consequently little chance of prestigious or well-paid employment. Girls will expect to move from dependence on their parents straight to dependence on their husbands.

Many studies describe this phenomenon and how, within the narrow confines of family life, women achieve status by producing children. A study of a small town community in Burkina Faso (*10*), for instance, showed the social dynamics at work behind the scenes. Less than one-third of the women had ever been to school, and less than 3% were wage-earners. Some kept up their traditional role of producing food, either on plots of land on the outskirts of town or by returning to their home villages, while others earned a little money buying and selling food in the market-place. In either activity, mothers were sharing the household duties, such as washing clothes, cooking and collecting water and firewood, with their children, who were sometimes sent to work for money themselves in the market or by watching over cars in town. The earnings of the women and their children were spent, by traditional division of responsibilities, on clothes and on special foods to supplement the basic diet.

The researchers found that within the sphere of home and housekeeping—but *only* within this sphere—women had complete authority, and children obviously increased the scope of their activities and their power. Furthermore, women in this society reached their highest status within the family when their own children married, because as mothers-in-law they were entitled to retire from work and devote themselves to their own concerns. "Under a system of this kind," concluded the study, "women with a large number of children gain both influence and prestige. By comparison, childless women are outsiders, they have no role in society, lack any authority and are pitied by all."

However, the researchers uncovered a paradox central to this discussion of how the status of women affects maternal mortality. Though the women in Burkina Faso were well aware of the fact that large families brought them prestige, they also knew from deep experience that constant child-bearing was exhausting and tied them to the treadmill of domesticity, and they expressed resentment. Thus "the very condition of high fertility that conferred prestige upon the women also proved to be the cause of their second-class status and of their dissatisfaction."

A study of women of the Patel caste in Rajasthan (*11*) gives another example of childbearing as the only path to fulfilment for women. It describes how custom and rigid tradition limit the communication a young bride can have with other members of her marital household (into which she has been bought by the payment of bride-price) until she has proved herself by bearing several children. Only 3% of the 168 women in the sample had ever been to school and most joined their marital home at around the age of 14 years. Furthermore, these young wives were at their least influential within the family during their most fertile years, so opportunities to plan their families would be practically non-existent.

## Virility—or machismo

In many societies, a wife who bears many children increases the status of her husband by constantly proving his virility. In some societies—notably in South America—this is prized so highly that it distorts the equation of desired family size and condemns many women to endless pregnancy for symbolic reasons alone. "The village would laugh at my husband if I didn't have a child every other year," explained one woman. And where the village is the setting for the whole of a person's life it is often not worth risking such scorn.

The effect of *machismo*, or the display of virility, on contraceptive practice will be discussed in the chapter on family planning. But where real communication between husband and wife is kept to a minimum—as for instance in polygamous societies—the tendency of men to see their families as instruments of their own aggrandizement is strongest and most difficult to challenge. Where husband and wife suffer together the consequences of over-large families, *machismo* is more easily recognized as a problem. But nowhere has it proved an easy attitude to dispel.

## Son preference

Another cause of high fertility directly associated with the status of women is the high value accorded to male children compared with female, which encourages women to go on bearing children until they have the desired number of sons (see Table 4.1).

Table 4.1. Preference for the sex of children

| Country | Index of son preference[a] | Country | Index of son preference[a] |
|---|---|---|---|
| **Strong son preference** | | **No preference** | |
| Pakistan | 4.9 | Guyana | 1.1 |
| Nepal | 4.0 | Indonesia | 1.1 |
| Bangladesh | 3.3 | Kenya | 1.1 |
| Republic of Korea | 3.3 | Peru | 1.1 |
| Syrian Arab Republic | 2.3 | Trinidad and Tobago | 1.1 |
| Jordan | 1.9 | Colombia | 1.0 |
| | | Costa Rica | 1.0 |
| **Moderate son preference** | | Ghana | 1.0 |
| Egypt | 1.5 | Panama | 1.0 |
| Lesotho | 1.5 | Paraguay | 1.0 |
| Senegal | 1.5 | Portugal | 1.0 |
| Sri Lanka | 1.5 | Haiti | 0.9 |
| Sudan | 1.5 | Philippines | 0.9 |
| Thailand | 1.4 | | |
| Turkey | 1.4 | **Daughter preference** | |
| Fiji | 1.3 | Venezuela | 0.8 |
| Nigeria | 1.3 | Jamaica | 0.7 |
| Tunisia | 1.3 | | |
| Yemen Arab Republic | 1.3 | | |
| Cameroon | 1.2 | | |
| Dominican Republic | 1.2 | | |
| Côte d'Ivoire | 1.2 | | |
| Malaysia | 1.2 | | |
| Mexico | 1.2 | | |
| Morocco | 1.2 | | |

[a] Index of son preference = Ratio of the number of mothers who prefer the next child to be male to the number of mothers who prefer the next child to be female.

Source: The health implications of sex discrimination in childhood. Unpublished document WHO/UNICEF/FHE/86.2.

Proverbs and sayings from many cultures indicate the pervasiveness and long-standing of son preference. An old proverb from China, for instance, says: "Eighteen goddess-like daughters are not equal to one son with a hump" (12). And among the Iteso of Uganda a newborn baby boy is described as "the central pole", indicating the central support of a spreading family, while a baby girl is described as "only

a prostitute" because her destiny is to be "sold" into
marriage in exchange for cattle (*13*).

Though son preference is primarily an attitude of mind, it is
both encouraged and reinforced by the patterns of society.
For instance, in most areas of the developing world the
family line is carried on through the sons, and there are
various restrictions on the right of females to inherit. Under
Islamic law, which operates mainly in parts of the Eastern
Mediterranean area, North Africa and Asia, a daughter
inherits only half of what a son inherits, and a widow is
entitled to only one-eighth of her husband's estate if she has
children and one-quarter if she is childless (*14*). Women in
the Philippines must seek the permission of their husbands to
acquire land. In traditional African societies land is appor-
tioned by tribal authorities to families according to how many
sons there are (*4*), and in Nepal only sons have the right to
inherit a leasehold title granted to a father (*15*).

Though bias in the rules of inheritance is now against the
law in many countries (in India, for example, the equal
rights of sons and daughters to inherit is enshrined in the
Constitution), it persists because of age-old tradition and the
powerlessness of dependent and often uneducated women to
demand their share.

In some parts of the world son preference is reinforced by
the practice of "dowry", in which a daughter ostensibly takes
with her at marriage her portion of the family's wealth. The
custom today is far removed from its original purpose, and
the parents of daughters are honour-bound to give as
generous a dowry as possible. Thus daughters become a
financial burden on their families, and where this custom
prevails, stories of poor families heavily in debt to local
money-lenders are common.

The sense that a daughter is a burden is enhanced by the
fact that her duty when she marries will be to her marital
home, and she will not even contribute to the support of her
parents when they are old. Sons, on the other hand, are seen
as an asset in such societies because they are expected to
find work later that will benefit their families, and to
strengthen the family unit through marriage.

Religion, too, has a part to play in son preference, though
this is often through a misinterpretation of original teachings
to give sex discrimination a bogus moral authority. In Hindu

religion only a son can perform the funeral rites for the father, and an orthodox Hindu who has only daughters risks being reborn as a lower form of life (*12*). Where Islamic tradition keeps women behind the veils of purdah and strongly restricts their movement in society, they must rely throughout life on men for support. This will be first their fathers, then their husbands, and if a woman should be widowed or divorced only her sons will give her security.

Because of the benefits that sons alone can bring, some women will go on trying for a son no matter how many daughters they have in the meantime. A cross-national survey in Asia found that a third of rural families in the Philippines, nearly a half in Thailand, and two-fifths in the Republic of Korea would go on having children until they produced a son, and others would only stop trying after they had produced three or four daughters in succession (*17*).

## Children as labour and security in old age

One of the most important reasons for women having many children is not connected with either their own prestige or their need for sons, but is to do with survival. In millions of poor families children are labour power.

The majority of the world's families still collect their basic needs—water, fuel, food—from their environment and the time taken just in running the household can be considerable. In one region of the Himalayas, for instance, women spend on average 7 hours on each of three days out of four gathering firewood, walking some 10 kilometres on each trip, to return bent under 25-kg loads (*18*). In Burkina Faso one study found women sleeping overnight at the distant water-hole that was their only source of supply. For all of these women there was still food to prepare at home, clothes to wash, children and old people to look after, and perhaps livestock to tend. A study in Rwanda found that daughters were shouldering about 40% of these responsibilities for their mothers.[1]

Besides such time-consuming household duties, poor families must support themselves either by cultivating their own plots of land, or by earning a living through productive

---

[1] *World survey: women in agriculture. Paper presented at the international conference to mark the end of the Women's Decade, Nairobi, 1985.* Unpublished United Nations document A/Conf. 1 16/4.

employment. Under such circumstances children are an asset as soon as they can shoulder some of the burden.

In Latin America the families with the most children are found among farm labourers. On the coffee and peanut plantations, for instance, children's nimble fingers at weeding- and picking-time can make the difference between a 10- and a 15-hour day for their parents.

In 1979 the International Labour Office (ILO) estimated that 55 million children around the world were at work helping to support their families, and other surveys have confirmed children's importance in this role. In one, 72% of people questioned in Mexico said they wanted children for economic support (*19*), and in another, 60% of rural Thais cited economic benefit as being the major advantage of having children (*17*).

In addition to the contribution many make while they are small, children also represent a source of security to their parents in old age. It is estimated that on average only 5% of the gross national product in developing countries is spent on social security, compared with 15% in Europe (*12*), and this benefits almost exclusively those in formal employment. By the year 2000 only 23% of men and 6% of women who are earning wages are likely to be eligible for pensions,[1] which means that the vast majority of people must make their own provision for old age. The Asian cross-national survey quoted above found that between 62% and 90% of poor urban and rural people would rely on their children to provide for them.

## Survival of children and family size

High fertility also goes hand in hand with high infant mortality. In poor regions of the world disease and hunger still carry off an average of one child in three during the most vulnerable years from birth to five years. Where the death of a child is a common event, parents will have large families simply because they do not expect all their children to survive, and this fatalistic attitude is reflected in folklore. "The first two are for the crows", says an Iranian proverb, and a Chinese saying goes, "One son is no son, two sons are an undependable son, and only three sons can be counted a real son" (*12*).

---

[1] *Information pack, World Assembly on Ageing, Vienna, 1982.* United Nations document.

## Teenage marriage

Teenage marriage, which is a reflection of the low status of women, is another social custom favouring high fertility. It is also a crucial factor in maternal mortality because of the number of years of childbearing ahead of the young bride, and because of the particular risk she runs in giving birth before she is fully developed.

The roots of teenage marriage are often buried deep in tradition, and in some countries, changing the legal age of marriage has been less successful in weeding it out than changing the prospects of women's lives through economic development. Thus in Sri Lanka, where the legal age of marriage for girls is 12 but the female literacy rate in 1971 was 70%, only 16% of girls are married while still in their teens.

Teenage marriage is widespread in the developing world, with the highest incidence in Bangladesh, where 72% of women aged 15–19 are married. For South Asia as a whole the percentage is 54%, compared with 24% for South-East Asia, 44% for Africa and 16% for Latin America (20).

In general, teenage marriage is more common in rural areas than in urban, reflecting the stronger adherence to tradition in remote communities rather than any practical difference. Its causes are intimately tied up with the image of ideal womanhood. Thus where a woman is seen primarily as wife and mother, there are benefits in starting to mould her personality to suit her husband and his family as early as possible. On the other side of the coin, where daughters are considered a financial burden on their own families, there is every incentive to be free of that burden as quickly as possible. Daughters are brought up as transitory members of the family, and a researcher in Bangladesh found the parents of a 12-year old bride very positive about this line of reasoning: "They felt that girls are born to be married and have children. They are not required to earn for the family, nor to look after the parents in their old age. Therefore, why should the parents waste money looking after them?" (21).

Other reasons for very early marriage relate to female sexuality, the need for men in a male-dominated society to control it, and the terrible stigma attached to pregnancy outside marriage. This has been dressed up in various beliefs and customs. Islamic law favours marriage at puberty, and in societies where girls generally marry very young, doubts about their "purity" grow with each year they remain unmarried after this milestone has been reached. In parts of India, dowry payments increase yearly from menarche onwards, "itself a sign that an unwed girl who has attained puberty can already be classed as damaged goods" (22). Furthermore, she may be prohibited from agricultural work from that point until she is married, thus increasing her burden on her family severalfold.

The overwhelming importance of sexual purity and fidelity to the husband in some cultures is demonstrated by the fact that obstructed labour is viewed as a sign that the woman has been unfaithful. In the midst of her agony she may be removed to a secluded place and left until she confesses her wrong-doing, gives birth or dies.[1]

## Education

Because high fertility is a feature of lack of choice or self-determination in women's lives, education has a dramatic effect on this picture, and therefore on maternal mortality.

Studies from many developing countries reveal that, as a general rule, the number of children a woman bears declines as her level of education rises. Thus in Colombia and the Sudan, women with 7 years' schooling are likely to have only half the number of children of their uneducated sisters. And women with secondary education in countries as diverse as Bangladesh, Kenya and Mexico are more than four times as likely to use contraceptives as women who have no education (2).

A survey of opinion on family planning in Jordan in 1972 revealed that 80% of those who disapproved of it were illiterate, 16% had received only primary education and 0.6% had received secondary education. None of the women who had attended university disapproved of family planning (23).

Here, access to information and a broadened understanding of the issue had a direct effect. However, the link between education and fertility is rarely so straightforward. Rather, education exerts its influence indirectly by raising the social status and self-image of women, by increasing their choices in

---

[1] *Traditional birth practices.* Unpublished document WHO/MCH/85.11.

life, and also their ability to question the status quo, make decisions for themselves and voice an opinion.

A project in Bangladesh, for instance, which gave daughters of marginal farmers the chance to go to school, reported dramatic changes in the lives of the girls, 95% of whom managed to stay in school for the five years of primary education. "Not one of them will marry a man she has not seen. The age of marriage has moved up, and they are definitely not having a baby in the first year of marriage," said the project's director (24).

The World Fertility Survey found that, in 10 of 14 developing countries, women with 7 or more years of schooling tended to marry an average of 3.5 years later than those with none (2).

But though education of girls is bound to undermine the tradition of child and teenage marriage and thereby affect the size of families and maternal mortality, it is also true that where the custom has deep roots there is resistance to education for girls because independent minds are not an asset. Thus teenage marriage and poor educational levels for girls are often found to reinforce each other.

## "Medication against fatalism"

Education has been described as "medication against fatalism". Certainly illiterate women are often found to have little understanding of the physiology of reproduction or how it can be altered, and to accept pregnancy as divinely ordained. This has a bearing on maternal mortality too, in that an uneducated woman will be susceptible to irrational explanations and dangerous interference for complications in pregnancy and childbirth.

For example, "gishiri cuts", a traditional surgical operation among the Hausa people of Nigeria, are commonly performed on uneducated women, while educated women rarely allow themselves to be subjected to this practice. The "gishiri cut" is a treatment for obstructed childbirth, and involves the cutting of the vagina by an elderly woman using an unsterilized blade.[1] African women coordinating the international campaign against female circumcision report that the custom is far more easily abolished among women with

---

[1] *Traditional birth practices.* Unpublished document WHO/MCH/85.11.

education who can question tradition than among those who are illiterate.

An uneducated woman is less ready to seek professional health care than her educated sister, either because she is not fully aware of what it has to offer or because she is frightened and out of her depth in the alien world of the health services.

Areas with the lowest female literacy rates frequently correspond to areas where fewest births are attended by trained personnel (see Table 4.2), and at least part of the explanation is the propensity of the mother to seek professional care. An analysis of maternal deaths in one Nigerian study, for instance, revealed that 219 of the 7654 women in the sample who had not received prenatal care died in childbirth compared with 19 of the 15 020 who had done so, and found that the most important influence on seeking prenatal care was education. Over 90% of the women in the survey who had received even as little as primary schooling had sought prenatal care (4).

Education works as "medication against fatalism" too in that the girl who has been educated has opened her mind to new ideas and the possibility of change. Kathleen Newland of the Worldwatch Institute describes well the potential of school to affect a girl's self-image: "For many women and girls, the classroom is the first and perhaps the only setting in which they perform as individuals rather than as members of a particular family, and the only context in which they can achieve a sense of worth and identity that does not come from their role as wives, mothers or daughters. In this, the school serves not only as a source of new knowledge about the world outside their immediate communities, but as a source of new knowledge about themselves as well" (23).

Depending on the conservatism of her community, an educated girl's world need not be the same as that of her mother and grandmother before her, and she may be able to find fulfilment through something other than motherhood.

## A passport to employment

The chance of finding employment outside the home—and outside the poorly paid, insecure and often exploitative world of casual work—is improved by education, and gets better the higher up the educational ladder a woman climbs.

Table 4.2. Global health for all and other indicators relating to women, health and development (about 1982)

| Region | WHO Global Indicators | | | | Others | | | | |
|---|---|---|---|---|---|---|---|---|---|
| | % adults who are literate (male/female) | % births attended by trained personnel | % infants with low birth weight | Infant mortality rate (male/female) | % enrolled in school | | | % women aged 15–19 who are married | Number of children per woman |
| | | | | | Ages 6–11 (male/female) | Ages 12–17 (male/female) | | | |
| WORLD | 67/54 | 56 | 16 | 103/92 | 76/64 | 55/46 | | 30 | 3.8 |
| Developed | 98/97 | 98 | 7 | 24/18 | 94/94 | 84/85 | | 8 | 2.0 |
| Developing | 52/32 | 49 | 18 | 116/104 | 70/53 | 42/28 | | 39 | 4.4 |
| AFRICA | 33/15 | 33 | 14 | 151/129 | 59/43 | 39/24 | | 44 | 6.4 |
| Northern | 44/18 | 30 | 10 | 128/114 | 70/45 | 42/43 | | 34 | 6.2 |
| Western | 20/6 | 39 | 17 | 171/145 | 44/30 | 29/16 | | 70 | 6.8 |
| Eastern | 29/14 | 26 | 13 | 142/121 | 55/41 | 33/20 | | 32 | 6.6 |
| Middle | 35/9 | 24 | 16 | 181/153 | 78/54 | 52/26 | | 49 | 6.0 |
| Southern | 55/56 | 66 | 12 | 109/92 | 82/86 | 74/70 | | 2 | 5.2 |
| NORTH AMERICA | 99/39 | 100 | 7 | 16/12 | 99/99 | 95/95 | | 11 | 1.8 |
| LATIN AMERICA | 76/70 | 65 | 10 | 90/80 | 78/78 | 58/54 | | 16 | 4.5 |
| Middle | 75/67 | 49 | 12 | 76/67 | 84/83 | 58/46 | | 21 | 5.3 |
| Caribbean | 67/66 | 60 | 12 | 78/68 | 85/87 | 60/59 | | 19 | 3.8 |
| Tropical South | 74/67 | 70 | 9 | 104/92 | 70/72 | 56/54 | | 15 | 4.6 |
| Temperate South | 93/91 | 88 | 7 | 47/41 | 98/98 | 70/73 | | 10 | 2.9 |
| ASIA | 56/34 | 51 | 20 | 108/99 | 73/54 | 43/28 | | 42 | 3.9 |
| South-West | 53/31 | 51 | 7 | 123/99 | 78/57 | 54/32 | | 25 | 5.8 |
| Middle South | 44/17 | 24 | 31 | 138/135 | 70/44 | 35/17 | | 54 | 5.5 |
| South-East | 75/53 | 52 | 17 | 105/87 | 71/65 | 43/35 | | 24 | 4.7 |
| East | 97/92 | 94 | 6 | 57/45 | 99/99 | 85/80 | | 2 | 2.3 |
| EUROPE | 96/93 | 97 | 7 | 25/19 | 95/96 | 81/80 | | 7 | 2.0 |
| Northern | 99/99 | 100 | 6 | 15/11 | 98/98 | 82/83 | | 9 | 1.8 |
| Western | 98/98 | 100 | 5 | 17/13 | 95/96 | 87/89 | | 5 | 1.6 |
| Eastern | 97/92 | 99 | 8 | 30/21 | 92/91 | 80/81 | | 9 | 2.3 |
| Southern | 93/85 | 93 | 7 | 31/25 | 97/97 | 73/66 | | 7 | 2.3 |
| USSR | 100/100 | | 8 | 35/27 | 99/99 | 72/82 | | 10 | 2.4 |
| OCEANIA | 90/88 | | 12 | 48/39 | 88/87 | 75/71 | | 10 | 2.8 |

Source: reference 20.

Figures from one study in Brazil, for instance, show that the chance of joining the formal labour force is twice as high for women who have completed primary school as for those with no schooling, and more than eight times as high for those who have completed secondary school (*14*).

An analysis of education levels and participation in the labour force in developing countries in the 1960s showed that over four times as many women with secondary education as with primary education had managed to secure formal employment outside agriculture in Egypt, the Syrian Arab Republic and Turkey (*25*). Where education offers the opportunity for this kind of employment there is an incentive for a woman to limit her family and, as a general rule, countries with a high proportion of women in the formal labour force are also countries with low birth rates.

Education plays an important part in this equation because it seems that it is not just having a job *per se* that influences a woman to limit her family, but the degree to which her work offers an alternative route to status and fulfilment. Where women's work outside the home is a matter of necessity and carries neither status nor security nor good pay, the link between employment and smaller families is not consistent. In India, for example, where the birth rate is high, 94% of working women are employed in the lowly paid and insecure informal sector (*16*).

## The privilege of the few

The greater opportunity education gives a girl to control her destiny and modify her role as a wife and mother is still denied to vast numbers. Female illiteracy has been described by UNESCO as an endemic problem in three-quarters of the world.

It is estimated that 68% of women in the developing world are illiterate, the rate of illiteracy being highest in Africa at 85% (compared to 67% for men), and lowest in Latin America at 30%. Furthermore, though 65% of girls of the appropriate age in developing countries were enrolled in primary school in 1985, the figure for secondary schools was only 37%, and for higher education, 10%.

These averages mask huge variations. As a general rule, and for a variety of reasons, rural people have higher levels of illiteracy than do urban people. Thus the 1981 Census for

India showed that the rate of literacy among the 214 million women who lived in the countryside was 18% compared with 48% for the 73 million women living in towns (*16*).

The drop-out rate, too, is far higher among country pupils than among city pupils in all areas. Just how dramatic the difference can be is demonstrated by the case of Guatemala, where studies show that only 4% of rural children complete primary school as against 50% of town children (*12*). Primary school drop-outs may not benefit even from the short time they spend in school since at least four or five years are considered necessary to ensure that the ability to read and write stays with a person for life.

Education is very much tied up with social status. Not surprisingly, people living in the poorest communities have the poorest educational status. But even within poor communities some people are more disadvantaged than others, as discrimination creeps into the equation too. Indian statistics, for example, show that illiteracy is particularly concentrated among the unscheduled castes and women of all castes.

Though poverty and underdevelopment mean that vast numbers of boys and girls never see the inside of a classroom, the greater disadvantage of women in education is universal in the developing countries. This both reflects and perpetuates their low status.

In Burkina Faso, where girls traditionally start work alongside their mothers at home and in the fields at the age of 7, while their brothers are not expected to contribute before they reach 11 years, boys outnumber girls in school by two to one.[1]

Girls in traditional Muslim homes whose freedom of movement and association is strictly limited, particularly after they reach puberty, may not be allowed to go to school if it is coeducational or if there are male teachers. In the Yemen Arab Republic, for instance, boys in school outnumber girls by seven to one. And in Bangladesh, teenage boys are six times more likely to be in school than girls, though at primary level the ratio of boys to girls is less than two to

---

[1] *World survey: women in agriculture. Paper presented at the international conference to mark the end of the Women's Decade, Nairobi, 1985.* Unpublished United Nations document A/Conf. 1 16/4.

one (*14*). In many places where girls marry very young, their position as schoolgirl is not in keeping with their position as wife and daughter-in-law, and their freedom of movement may be curtailed.

In other circumstances girls are not sent to school because parents do not expect to benefit from it. Daughters are not expected to support themselves or their aged parents later in life, and any benefit that does arise from education will be reaped by their marital households. Pressure against educating daughters will be particularly strong in families that depend on the labour or earnings of their children to survive. If sacrifices have to be made to allow their children to go to school, parents will favour their sons in the hope that the investment will pay off in better employment later on.

"Illiteracy is a personal tragedy, and a powerful force in preserving inequalities and oppression," writes the sociologist Paul Harrison (*12*). But where discrimination is rooted deep in society, illiteracy proves difficult to tackle even with well-intentioned laws. Under the Indian Constitution, for example, primary schooling is compulsory for boys and girls, yet it is estimated that only 22% of all girls between 11 and 14 years of age are beneficiaries of the minimum formal education that is their right (*16*).

Many people believe education is the key to improving the status of women, and that a great many evils suffered by them at the moment would be swept away by the tide of universal formal schooling. As far as maternal death is concerned, the evidence is there that education plays a powerful role, and there is now an urgent need for more research to establish the links more clearly.

## Health

The link between the general health status of women and maternal mortality is already clear. A woman whose growth is stunted from malnutrition and who is debilitated by anaemia and long hours of hard physical work each day will start the demanding process of pregnancy already in poor condition. If complications occur, her chances of surviving, even with professional help, will be lessened.

In the developing world (excluding China) an estimated 25% of city dwellers and 71% of rural people are without safe drinking-water, and 47% and 87% of urban and rural people, respectively, have no access to proper sanitation (20). Such conditions of poverty and underdevelopment threaten the health of the whole community—men, women and children. But because of the additional effects of sex discrimination the dice are loaded more heavily against females.

Sex discrimination acts on the health of women in a number of ways: through differential feeding, through the so-called "double day" in which women working outside the home are also expected to run their households, and through the lack of provision for their special needs in the health services.

## Less food for females

Many of the health problems that affect women in their childbearing years have their roots in childhood. As has already been seen, the preference for sons is widespread in the developing world, and though of itself this need not be harmful, evidence suggests that son preference usually goes hand in hand with neglect of daughters.

During childhood boys and girls require, on a weight-for-weight basis, equal amounts of all nutrients. Yet in very many places girls receive less from the family pot than their brothers. A study carried out in 1981 in a group of villages in Bangladesh found that, up to the age of 5 years, the calorie intake of girls was on average 16% less than that of boys, and the discrepancy was 11% for the age group 5–14 years. As a result, 14% of the female children in the survey were severely malnourished compared with 5% of the male children, and 26% of the girls were severely stunted compared with 18% of the boys (26). In Mexico, too, a study in the state of Tlaxcala found that the girls received less than the boys of all the nutrients monitored (27).

Less direct discrimination against infant girls has been described in Uttar Pradesh, India (28). Researchers carrying out a field study found that women anxious for sons would aim to become pregnant again as soon as possible if the first child was a daughter, and that they would stop breast-feeding the baby girl as soon as they became pregnant. If, on the other hand, the first child was a son, they would try to delay another pregnancy as long as possible, and would breast-feed for an extended period to give the baby a sound start in life.

The study also found that, while children were growing up, boys were given more of the "rich" foods like milk, butter and eggs than their sisters. It was deemed important that boys, who would support their families later on, should grow up big and strong and they were therefore given the lion's share of the most nutritious foods. But parents were reluctant anyway to give their daughters much of these foods because they believed that a high-calorie diet would hasten puberty and thereby saddle them prematurely with the burden of dowry. This may offer a clue to why, even in better-off households where food is reasonably plentiful, girls are still frequently less well nourished than their brothers in many parts of the developing world.

This phenomenon is demonstrated starkly in a study from West Bengal, India, in which the nutritional status of children in two villages—Sahajapur and Kuchli—was compared. Whereas girls were found to be 4% more undernourished than boys in Sahajapur, the figure for Kuchli was much higher, at 41%, despite the fact that there were more landless families and lower nutritional standards overall in Sahajapur than in Kuchli. The conclusion was that land reform and the higher nutritional standards it encouraged among the families of Kuchli had benefited only the boys, whose nutritional status improved enormously, while for their sisters little changed (29).

If girls do not get adequate supplies of protein, calcium and vitamin D while they are developing, their bones do not grow as long and strong as they should, and the consequent stunting of these children makes them particularly vulnerable to difficulties in labour. In Zaria, Northern Nigeria, it is estimated that 25% of the childbearing population are stunted in this way (4). But sex bias in the distribution of food within families does not only affect girls as they grow up. It is the custom in many societies for adult women, together with young children, to eat after the men have had their fill, with the result that they tend to get less of the more nutritious foods. A survey of 898 villages throughout the world found it to be a general rule that the needs of the men were given priority at mealtimes (30).

Surveys have also found that women are most affected by cultural food taboos, many of which are related to pregnancy.

# MATERNAL MORTALITY RATES
## Range per 100,000 live births

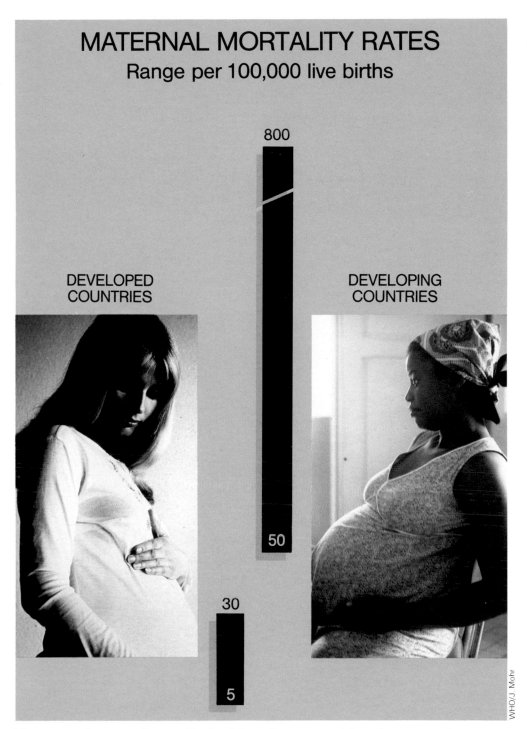

800

DEVELOPED
COUNTRIES

DEVELOPING
COUNTRIES

50

30

5

WHO/J. Mohr

**The rates of maternal mortality in rich and poor countries show a greater disparity than any other public health indicator.**

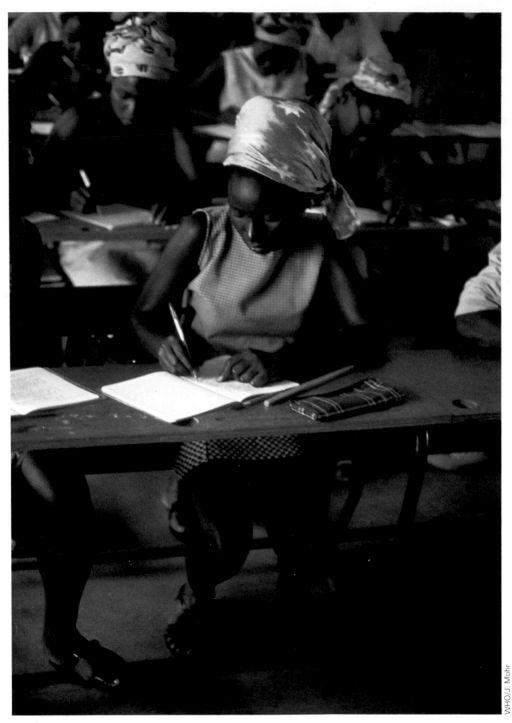

**"Medication against fatalism"** – education is seen by many as the key to improving the status of women.

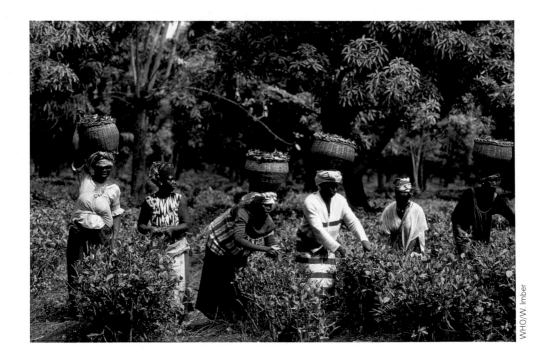

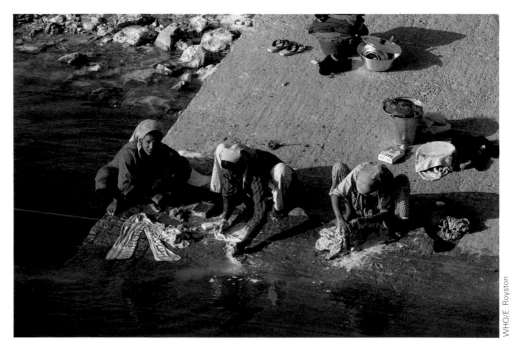

**Many women carry a double burden – helping to support the family by working outside the home and taking full responsibility for housekeeping and child care.**

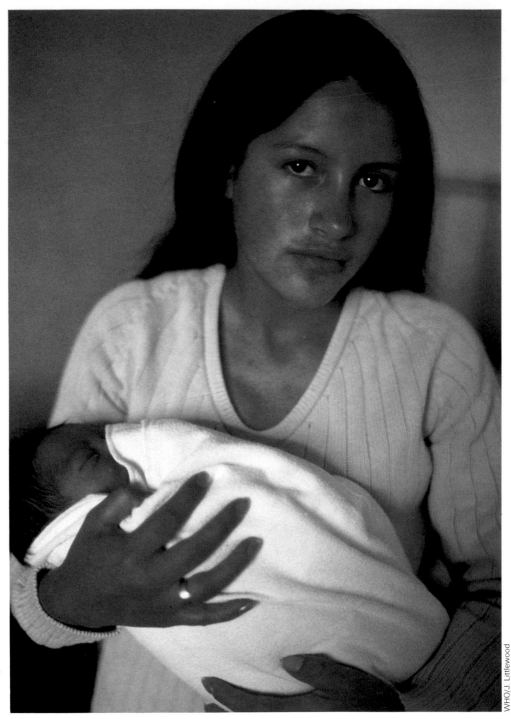

**Early marriage and childbearing are common in many countries, often setting the scene for high fertility and correspondingly high maternal mortality.**

In Ethiopia and the Sudan for instance, pregnant women
are given low-calorie food to prevent the fetus from growing
too big and causing difficulties in labour. And in northern
Nigeria different groups observe different taboos for pregnant
women, ranging from the avoidance of various fruits and
vegetables, popularly believed to cause neonatal jaundice
and worm infestation, to avoidance of rice, thought to cause
boils and skin diseases, and milk, thought to cause a vaginal
discharge that harms the eyes of the newborn baby.[1] The
food restrictions in Nigeria are removed as soon as the woman
gives birth and she is encouraged to eat more protein and
high-calorie foods and to rest if possible.

As was discussed earlier, many societies either do not
recognize or simply cannot meet the extra nutritional and
rest requirements of pregnant and lactating women. Here
again the status of women will play a part, dictating whether
or not other family members are prepared to give a mother's
needs priority over their own.

## Odds against survival

In many places the neglect of girls does not stop at
inadequate feeding; there is overwhelming evidence that they
are also given less care and attention during sickness than
their brothers. One study in India, for example, found that
boys admitted to hospital suffering from protein-energy
malnutrition (PEM) outnumbered girls by between 47 and 53
to one, though the condition was four or five times more
common among girls in the research area (31). And a study
in Bangladesh found that though equal proportions of girls
and boys were afflicted with diarrhoea, 66% more boys than
girls were taken to health facilities for treatment (32).

Similar stories come from other parts of the world where
daughters are less valued than sons. Some tell of parents
being prepared to spend money on treatment for their sons
that they would not spend on sick daughters; others of girls
not being immunized against childhood diseases at the same
rate as boys where the service is not free.

At its most extreme, this sex bias in feeding and care has
resulted in increased rates of female mortality in childhood,
and in some countries this has been sharp enough to lower

---

[1] *Traditional birth practices.* Unpublished document WHO/MCH/85.11.

the life expectancy of women, despite their natural propensity to outlive men.

Generally speaking, girls are born with a biological advantage over boys, which makes them more resistant to infection and malnutrition. So, where treatment is even-handed, girls should be at less risk of dying in their first five years of life than boys. The odds are 1.15:1 in favour of girls, but in a number of countries and on every continent the biological advantage of girls has been cancelled out by their social disadvantage (see Table 4.3). Field research has failed to establish firmly the cause of this unnatural imbalance in child mortality. However, the circumstantial evidence is over-whelming that discrimination is the crucial factor.

Table 4.3.   Ratio of mortality rates between males and females, for infants, toddlers and children

| Country[a] | Infant | Toddler[b] | Child[c] |
|---|---|---|---|
| India | 0.92 | —0.96— | |
| Senegal | 1.16 | 0.99 | 1.00 |
| Nepal | 1.03 | 0.89 | 0.95 |
| Bangladesh | 1.18 | 0.73 | 0.84 |
| Pakistan | 1.05 | 0.65 | 0.68 |
| Cameroon | 1.07 | 1.04 | 0.99 |
| Egypt | 1.01 | 0.71 | 0.94 |
| Turkey | 1.10 | 0.62 | 0.94 |
| Côte d'Ivoire | 1.24 | 1.19 | 1.11 |
| Indonesia | 1.30 | 1.15 | 1.31 |
| Morocco | 1.06 | 0.88 | 1.11 |
| Kenya | 1.10 | 1.17 | 1.02 |
| Ghana | 1.22 | 1.15 | 0.95 |
| Colombia | 1.19 | 0.75 | 0.83 |
| Tunisia | 1.02 | 1.05 | 1.25 |
| Mexico | 1.25 | 0.86 | 0.88 |
| Thailand | 1.08 | 1.42 | 0.65 |
| Syrian Arab Republic | 0.92 | 1.05 | 0.64 |
| Sri Lanka | 1.24 | 0.68 | 0.87 |
| Jordan | 0.85 | 0.81 | 0.99 |
| Venezuela | 1.27 | 1.14 | 0.90 |
| Fiji | 1.19 | 0.92 | 1.04 |
| Jamaica | 1.36 | 1.07 | 1.17 |
| Malaysia | 1.31 | 1.41 | 1.19 |
| Portugal | 1.49 | 1.52 | 0.59 |
| Sweden | 1.09 | —1.27— | |

[a] Countries are ordered by level of under-five mortality.
[b] Toddler: mortality between first and second birthdays.
[c] Child: mortality between second and fifth birthdays.

Source: Health implications of sex discrimination in childhood. Unpublished document WHO/UNICEF/FHE/86.2.

Furthermore, as a result of the extremely low status of women, imbalances in the rates of male and female mortality can persist well beyond the vulnerable first five years of life, and figures from censuses show that this has been the trend in India since 1951. By 1971, female mortality rates in India were higher than those for males for every year of life from one to 49, and life expectancy for women at birth was lower than that for men. Commenting on the figures, the sociologist Maitrayee Mukhopadhyay said: "One conclusion is inescapable; women's lives are cheaper and more expendable than men's. Their inferior status stands in the way of their survival" (*16*).

## A double day's work

Another factor in the equation of female health and survival is the number of hours a woman must work each day, and the kind of tasks she must perform. Much will depend on the economic circumstances of her life. Where people live in poverty, men, women and children have to work hard to survive, with little help from technology or modern services to lighten the workload.

During the UN Decade for Women attention was drawn to the fact that nearly everywhere women are bearing a double burden. While they are helping to support their families with work outside the home, they are, at the same time, carrying full responsibility for housekeeping and child care.

Until very recently this pattern was hidden so successfully behind the veil of familiarity and passive acceptance that women's real contribution to the economy did not appear in any conventional statistics. This applied not only to the labour required in fetching water, gathering firewood, preparing meals and supervising others who help with the household tasks, but also to vast amounts of agricultural labour done by women—largely because it, too, is unpaid, but also because some men are ashamed to admit that their wives work.

According to the Food and Agriculture Organization of the United Nations (FAO), women make up 47% of the agricultural labour force in Africa, 40% in Asia, 25% in North Africa and the Eastern Mediterranean region and 19% in Latin America (*33*). But these figures refer only to waged workers. Behind the scenes on all continents women are growing vegetables on patches of land, weeding, hoeing, transplanting seedlings, raising hens and tending livestock, either to produce food for their families or as free labour on their family farms. More realistic estimates of their contribution, therefore, suggest that, in the developing world, women produce at least half the world's food, and that they do 60–90% of agricultural work in Africa (*30*), 50% in Asia and nearly 50% in Latin America (*14*).

Partly because so much of their outside labour is unpaid and therefore "invisible", women are rarely relieved of any of their housekeeping responsibilities by their menfolk. "In most parts of India it is considered shameful for men to take part in household chores," says Maitrayee Mukhopadhyay, "and women working as farm labourers put in an average of 14 hours per day. This includes, besides the hard manual labour necessary in agriculture, arduous tasks like collecting firewood and transporting it from distant places, fetching water and trips to and from the fields to the house to cook and serve the food. Although male farm labourers also do heavy manual work it is limited to the work hours. On returning home they have leisure" (*16*).

Though there is evidence from some places that poverty breaks down the traditional divisions of labour, in most it does not, and the picture presented of India is repeated around the world. In rural Botswana, for instance, women work on average 7 hours a day and men 5 hours; and in rural Java the average figures are 11 hours and 8.5 hours respectively (*34*). Studies in Malaysia and the Philippines reveal that men devote nearly all their time to paid work, and that their small share of work in the home is only slightly affected by increases or decreases in the total burden of housework. For women, on the other hand, the workload changes constantly with the demands of raising children and seasonal work in agriculture (*34*).

Though many women accept a heavy burden of work and chronic fatigue as normal and inescapable, such a situation has far-reaching effects on their health. "It could perhaps be the contributing cause for the higher rates of female mortality in recent decades and the dwindling sex ratios," says a report from India (*16*). And a study from Burkina Faso indicates that during the rainy season, when work in the fields is heaviest, women are sometimes too tired at the end of the day to prepare a proper meal. As a result whole families are reported to lose weight at this time of the year (*14*).

As has been discussed earlier, the double workload is particularly threatening to the health of women who are pregnant or breast-feeding, and may affect the survival chances of mother and infant.

The blindness of conventional labour statistics to work that is not paid has had dire consequences for women in other ways too—particularly in the so-called development process. In effect it has set them on a downward spiral of deteriorating status and pushed them even further on to the unskilled, labour-intensive fringes of production.

In the Gambia, for instance, the rain-fed rice fields which produce 84% of the country's crop are cultivated by women, yet rain-fed cultivation is allocated less than 4% of the budget for rice projects (*33*). This is a common pattern in developing countries; though an estimated 85% of the female population overall works in agriculture, there are very few female agricultural advisers and, as a rule, skills training, land reform and loans favour men. Furthermore, the first operations to be mechanized are those done by men and, as can be seen from the case study of a family in India, this often adds to the workload of women. Here, a tractor was bought to help the men of the household with ploughing. As a result, they were able to increase the acreage under cultivation, but for the women who did the manuring, weeding, harvesting and threshing, the work was doubled, because not one of their operations was mechanized (*16*).

A twist in the story of mechanization is that when a task traditionally performed by women—such as milling or threshing—is mechanized, it is often taken over by men, and women have to look elsewhere for work. This process has run to extremes in Brazil, which has the most 'masculine' labour force in the world. A study of the labour market in that country shows how women have progressively been squeezed out by industrialization since the turn of the century (*34*). On the one hand, investment in more sophisticated technology has displaced them in factories, and on the other hand, where men have been drawn into new industries, women have been left to cultivate the land. In poor households women have no choice but to work, so the limiting of their opportunities to the more tedious, low-paid jobs is an unavoidable threat to their status.

Quite apart from any moral considerations, leaving women out of the equation is bound to hinder the progress of development sooner or later, and this fact is now dawning on governments. One aspect of development in which this is already apparent is the attempt to provide clean water and sanitation in Third World villages. Efforts have been constantly frustrated as water pumps have broken down faster than new ones are being installed and communities have been apathetic about the idea of latrines. This has particularly serious implications for health because some 80% of all illness in the world is thought to be caused by lack of clean water and sanitation.

Part of the reason for the slow progress is that, though women collect most of the water, few have been trained to maintain or mend pumps, and they must therefore rely on the goodwill of men to keep them in working order. Similarly with private latrines, women have most to gain from them because they are most inhibited by social taboos about defecating. Researchers in Bangladesh, for instance, found women preserving their modesty by relieving themselves only during the hours of darkness (and often having to endure "discomfort" during the day) (*18*), while in some Muslim countries women in purdah have to use the rooftops to defecate. In most places men are free from such inhibitions; sanitation is therefore a low priority for them, yet it is they who make the decisions and have to design and implement the community programmes.

As these examples show, the status of women affects their general health in many direct and indirect ways. But what is the picture of health care for women? How responsive is it to their needs, and how well do they use the services that are available?

## Health care for women

Every year there are some 500 000 maternal deaths and millions of women are seriously ill after giving birth. Yet nearly half the births in developing countries are not attended by trained health personnel. In Africa only 34% of mothers have trained attendants, while in South Asia the figure is 31% and in Latin America, 64%. Even fewer women receive prenatal care.

This is partly due to woeful inadequacies in provision; developing countries spend on average 2% of the gross national product on health services, with the result that many millions of people live beyond the reach of modern medicine. But it is also due to the fact that the services that do exist are not reaching women as they should.

In most developing countries good baseline data are not available to health planners. Yet services can only be truly effective when they are based, firstly, on an accurate picture of the health problems of people, and therefore their needs and, secondly, on an appreciation of the complex social, cultural and economic factors that affect use of health facilities. Availability of services does not, on its own, guarantee access.

This is probably more true for women than men because they are less autonomous, yet health planners tend to see users of health facilities as a homogeneous group. For them, meeting women's needs simply means providing special services such as maternal and child health care and family planning, not searching for answers to why women are less willing patients than men, and adapting the health system to give them better access, though both approaches are necessary.

Largely as a consequence of their low status, women face numerous barriers between themselves and the health services. As was discussed earlier, women without education are less ready than those who are literate to use modern facilities because such facilities are alien. Other possible reasons are that they are kept waiting a long time at clinics and then treated with disrespect by the staff. Younger women look to their elders for advice, and if humiliating treatment by health staff is a common experience women will not encourage each other to go for prenatal care even if it is available. And when labour starts a woman will turn most readily to the traditional midwife, whose face is familiar and comforting but who may use unhygienic methods that will pose a threat to her health.

In some parts of the world a woman cannot visit a clinic or hospital without the permission of her husband or mother-in-law. Where this tradition is strong, when the husband is away others may not be prepared to take the decision even on behalf of a woman suffering problems in labour.

Another common obstacle is the fact that health personnel are predominantly male. A woman may be extremely shy about being treated by a man, and there may also be strong cultural taboos. In India 90% of the community health workers—trained to deliver care at the village level where it is most appropriate for women—are men and the majority of their patients are also men. The original plan was to train mostly female community health workers, but the taboo against women being touched by men was not so simply bypassed and it inhibited women from coming forward for training (*35*).

For Indian women there is a stigma attached to being ill—it has overtones of not being able to cope as well as others—and they tend to ignore health problems until they can no longer keep going. In addition, poor women who are tied to long hours of work, child care and housekeeping find it hard to take time off to visit a clinic. They may forfeit much-needed wages; they may have no one immediately available to look after their children or take over vital household chores, and they may not have the fare for public transport.

The logistics of seeking treatment are particularly complicated for women the world over, yet few health services make this their concern. Indeed, in some places services are rigidly divided between preventive and curative care so that, for example, a woman cannot get medicines at the prenatal clinic but is sent elsewhere for supplies (*35*).

The fact that the health services in most countries are so poorly adapted to the needs of women is partly explained by their having a very small voice in the corridors of power; very few women are involved in management or decision-making in the health services.

Thus the low status of women is self-perpetuating. It will take enormous political will to break the cycle, but since the UN Decade for Women there are some hopeful signs that governments are taking more note of sex discrimination and its distorting effects in all areas of life.

For many women death in childbirth is the final, devastating signal of their low status. Pregnancy and childbirth will continue to take an unnecessarily high toll of life wherever discrimination against women systematically undermines their health and ignores their special needs for care. Addressing the "causes behind the causes" is therefore absolutely vital in any attempt to control maternal mortality. However, measures to improve social conditions for women must never be considered an alternative to professional maternity care but rather as complementing it. Though pregnancy is essentially a healthy process, unexpected complications occur even in the most healthy social environments, and at this point efficient medical services are absolutely necessary to save lives.

# References

1. LYONS, C. More than a medical issue. *Women's world*, **6**: 30–32 (1985).
2. WORLD FERTILITY SURVEY. *Fertility in the developing world.* Voorburg, Netherlands, 1984.
3. MOERMAN, M. L. Growth of the birth canal in adolescent girls. *American journal of obstetrics and gynecology*, **143**(5): 528–532 (1982).
4. HARRISON, K. A. Child bearing, health and social priorities. A survey of 22,774 consecutive births in Zaria, Northern Nigeria. *British journal of obstetrics and gynaecology*, Supplement No. 5 (1985).
5. WALKER, G. J. Maternal mortality in Jamaica. *Lancet,* **1**(8479): 486–488 (1986).
6. HARRINGTON, J. A. Nutritional stress and economic responsibility: a study of Nigerian women. In: Buvinic, M., ed., *Women and poverty in the Third World.* Baltimore, Johns Hopkins University Press, 1983.
7. ROYSTON, E. The prevalence of nutritional anaemia in women in developing countries: a critical review of available information. *World health statistics quarterly*, **35**: 52–91 (1982).
8. JIMENEZ HOUDEK, M. & NEWTON, N. Activities and work during pregnancy and the postpartum period: a cross-cultural study of 202 societies. *American journal of obstetrics and gynecology*, **135**: 171–176 (1979).
9. GREENWOOD, A. ET AL. A prospective study of pregnancy in a rural area of the Gambia, West Africa. *Bulletin of the World Health Organization*, **65**(5): 635–644 (1987).
10. VAN DE WALLE, F. & OUAIDOU, N. Status and fertility among urban women in Burkina Faso. *International family planning perspectives*, **11**(2): 60–64 (1985).
11. PATEL, T. Domestic group, status of women and fertility. *Social action*, **32**(4): 363–379 (1982).
12. HARRISON, P. *Inside the Third World.* London, Pelican, 1979.
13. AKELLO, G. Children that prove a woman's value. *People*, **10**(4): 3–5 (1983).
14. TAYLOR, D. *Women: world report.* London, Methuen, 1985.
15. STAUDT, K. The landless majority. *People*, **7**(3): 7 (1980).
16. MUKHOPADHYAY, M. *Silver shackles: women and development in India.* Oxford, Oxfam Publications, 1984.

17. ARNOLD, F. & KUO, E. C. Y. The value of daughters and sons: a comparative study of the gender preferences of parents. *Journal of comparative family studies,* **15**(2): 299–318 (1984).

18. AGARWAL, A. & ANAND, A. Ask the women who do the work. *New scientist,* **96**(1330): 302–304 (1982).

19. UNITED NATIONS FUND FOR POPULATION ACTIVITIES. *State of the world's population.* New York, 1983.

20. WORLD HEALTH ORGANIZATION. *Women, health and development: A report by the Director-General.* Geneva, 1985 (WHO Offset Publication, No. 90).

21. ISLAM, M. Child wives of Bangladesh. *People,* **12**(3): 8–9 (1985).

22. CALDWELL, J. C. ET AL. The causes of marriage change in south India. *Population studies,* **37**: 343–361 (1983).

23. NEWLAND, K. *Women and population growth. Choices beyond childbearing.* Washington, Worldwatch Institute, 1977.

24. ROWLEY, J. Can Bangladesh change the system? *People,* **12**(3): 10–13 (1985).

25. YOUSSEF, N. H. *Women and work in developing societies.* Berkeley, University of California, 1974 (Population Monograph No. 15).

26. CHEN, L. C. ET AL. Sex bias in the family allocation of food and health care in rural Bangladesh. *Population and development review,* **7**(1): 55–70 (1981).

27. PELTO, G. H. Intrahousehold food distribution patterns. In: *Malnutrition: determinants and consequences.* New York, Alan R. Liss, 1984.

28. KHAN, M. E. ET AL. *Health practices in Uttar Pradesh. A study of discrimination against women.* Baroda, Operations Research Group, 1985 (Working paper No. 45).

29. SEN, A. & SENGUPTA, S. Malnutrition of rural children and the sex bias. *Economic and political weekly,* **18**: 855–864 (1983).

30. SCHOFIELD, S. *Development and the problems of village nutrition.* London, Croom Helm, 1979.

31. GOPALAN, C. & NAIDU, A. N. Nutrition and fertility. *Lancet,* **2**(7786): 1077–1079 (1972).

32. SABIR, N. I. & EBRAHIM, G. J. Are daughters more at risk than sons in some societies? *Journal of tropical pediatrics,* **30**: 237–239 (1984).

33. FOOD AND AGRICULTURE ORGANIZATION OF THE UNITED NATIONS. *Women in agriculture, No. 1.* Rome, 1984.

34. BUVINIC, M. ET AL. *Women and poverty in the Third World.* Baltimore & London, Johns Hopkins University, 1983.

35. MURTHY, N. Reluctant patients—the women of India. *World health forum,* **3**(3): 315–316 (1982).

# Chapter 5

# CAUSES OF MATERNAL DEATH

It is customary to classify the causes of maternal deaths under three headings: direct, indirect and coincidental. Direct causes refer to diseases or complications that occur only during pregnancy, including abortion, ectopic pregnancy (a pregnancy that develops outside the uterus), hypertensive diseases of pregnancy, antepartum and postpartum haemorrhage, obstructed labour, and puerperal sepsis. Indirect causes are diseases that may be present before pregnancy but are aggravated by pregnancy; examples include heart disease, anaemia, essential hypertension (high blood pressure of unknown origin), diabetes mellitus and haemoglobinopathies (diseases of the red blood cells). Coincidental causes are fortuitous in nature; deaths from road traffic accidents are a typical example.

In fact, the reasons that women die in pregnancy and childbirth are many-layered. Behind the medical causes there are logistic causes—failures in the health care system, lack of transport, etc. These will be treated more fully in Chapter 8. And behind these are all the social, cultural and political factors which together determine the status of women, their health, fertility and health-seeking behaviour, and which form the subject of Chapter 4.

The direct causes together with anaemia are responsible for more than 80% of all maternal deaths reported from the Third World, and the picture is remarkably similar wherever rates of maternal mortality are high (see Table 5.1). In this chapter an account will be given of each of these diseases, its chief causes, the type of women most likely to be affected, and what can be done to prevent it. An outline of the treatment of each disease will also be presented.

## Hypertensive disease of pregnancy

This group of diseases includes pre-eclampsia and eclampsia. The characteristics of pre-eclampsia are high blood pressure, protein in the urine and swelling of the tissues (oedema)

## Table 5.1. Main causes of maternal deaths in hospitals in selected developing countries

| | India | Pakistan | Malaysia | Viet Nam | Indonesia | Islamic Republic of Iran | Fiji | Nigeria | Ghana | Malawi | Zimbabwe | Kenya | United Republic of Tanzania | Egypt |
|---|---|---|---|---|---|---|---|---|---|---|---|---|---|---|
| Haemorrhage | + | + | + | + | + | + | + | + | + | + | + | + | + | + |
| Sepsis | + | + | | | + | + | | + | + | + | + | + | + | + |
| Toxaemia | + | + | + | + | + | + | | + | + | + | + | | + | + |
| Abortion | | | | | | | + | | | | | | | + |
| Obstructed labour/ ruptured uterus | | + | | + | | | | + | + | + | + | + | + | |
| Hepatitis | + | | | | | + | + | | | | + | | | |
| Anaemia | + | + | | + | | | + | + | | | | | + | |
| Abnormal haemoglobin | | | + | | | | | | | | | | | |
| Cardiac diseases | | | | | | + | + | | | | | | | |
| *Source reference:* | *1* | *2* | *3* | *4* | *5* | *6* | *7* | *8, 9* | *10* | *11* | *12* | *13* | *14* | |

WHO document FHE/PMM/89.9.18

during the second half of pregnancy. In some cases, the condition remains mild throughout pregnancy. In others, it may become severe, with a further rise in the blood pressure and increase in the amount of protein in the urine. Headaches, vomiting, impairment of vision, and pain in the upper abdomen occur and the affected woman may then stop producing urine. In the last and most severe stage of this disease, convulsions develop; this is the stage referred to as eclampsia. If eclampsia is left untreated, the woman rapidly becomes unconscious and dies from heart failure, kidney failure, liver failure or brain haemorrhage. In tropical Africa the disease can develop rapidly, progressing from the earliest physical signs right through to eclampsia within 24 hours.[1] One group of researchers estimated that the average time between the onset of symptoms and death from this condition is two days.[2]

Pre-eclampsia, common during first pregnancies, is rare in subsequent pregnancies, except where the woman is very overweight, has diabetes mellitus or essential hypertension, or is expecting a multiple birth. For an unknown reason the incidence of pre-eclampsia in black people and Indians is higher than in white people, even allowing for differences in age, parity and living standards. The very young (that is, girls in the early teenage years who are pregnant for the first time), and those over the age of 35 years are particularly vulnerable. The condition affects all social classes equally but because the poor are sometimes unable to afford the cost of proper health care, or even because some poor people mistrust expert medical care and are reluctant to use it even when available, they are the ones most likely to develop eclampsia. There is also evidence that pre-eclampsia runs in families, the disease being more common in daughters of women who have themselves had pre-eclampsia.

The cause of pre-eclampsia is not known. Treatment is therefore aimed at relieving the symptoms and at ending the pregnancy as soon as the baby is considered able to survive. Bed rest is important, and sedative drugs are commonly prescribed. Drugs that lower the blood pressure also have their place. Some women with pre-eclampsia go into labour

---

[1] Lawson, J. B. *Childbirth in Africa.* Paper prepared for the WHO Regional Multidisciplinary Consultative Meeting on Human Reproduction, Yaoundé, 4–7 December 1978. Unpublished WHO document HRP/RMC/78.8.
[2] Maine, D. et al. *Prevention of maternal deaths in developing countries: program options and practical considerations.* Paper prepared for the International Safe Motherhood Conference, Nairobi, 10—13 February 1987.

spontaneously. For those who do not, the accepted practice is to induce labour at the 37th or 38th week of gestation; if subsequent progress is slow, or if conditions are unfavourable for induction, then the baby should be delivered by caesarean section.

Where the condition has developed into eclampsia, prompt treatment must be given if the mother is to survive. This disease carries a death rate of 5% or even higher. The main objectives of treatment are to control the convulsions and lower the blood pressure, and, once these have been achieved, to deliver the baby rapidly. Induction of labour is often necessary but for women who do not deliver within 6 hours of the start of treatment, a caesarean section must be undertaken if the mother is to have a chance of survival. Measures to prevent further convulsions should continue after delivery. For the following 48 hours, injections of very potent sedative drugs will ensure that the patient remains semiconscious. Meanwhile, nourishment can be maintained by the use of glucose solutions administered through continuous intravenous drip. Throughout this period, maternal survival depends largely on skilled nursing care.

Prenatal care can greatly improve the chances of detecting pre-eclampsia early. If expectant mothers pay weekly visits to the prenatal clinic during the last 4–6 weeks of pregnancy, the opportunity can be taken to test their urine for protein, measure their blood pressure and search for signs of oedema. The detection of pre-eclampsia is an indication that the mother should be referred to hospital for delivery. However, in parts of the world where women do not have access to prenatal care that can warn them of the risks in advance, or trained attendants during childbirth, or speedy access to a hospital when emergencies occur, pregnancy hypertension (or toxaemia) may account for a high proportion of deaths. In community studies it was found to be the single most important direct obstetric cause of maternal mortality in Jamaica (15), accounting for 26% of such deaths; second only to abortion as a cause of death in Cali, Colombia,[1] accounting for about 34% of direct obstetric deaths; and the cause of between 15% and 21% of such deaths in Bangladesh (16). Furthermore, a survey of maternal deaths in Menoufia, Egypt, and Bali, Indonesia found that women

[1] Rodriguez, J. et al. Avoidable mortality and maternal mortality in Cali, Colombia. In: *Interregional Meeting on the Prevention of Maternal Mortality, Geneva, 11–15 November 1985.* Unpublished WHO document FHE/PMM/85.9.1.

under 20 years old were 3 times (in Menoufia) and 4.8 times (in Bali) more likely to die of this cause than older women (*17*).

Data from Sweden reveal how important early detection of toxaemia is in saving lives (*18*). In the period 1950–55 about 14% of pregnant women suffering from this condition died compared with only 3% in 1971–80, though the incidence of the disease did not alter significantly, nor did the proportion of women delivering their babies in hospital. The steep decline in the case–fatality rate was the result of better prenatal care and treatment of women with early signs of toxaemia.

## Obstructed labour and rupture of the uterus

The incidence of obstructed labour varies considerably between countries. A study in Cameroon[1] found the condition in 3.5% of deliveries, as compared with 2.3% in a Brazilian study (*19*), and between 5.8% and 13.5% in several studies from South-East Asian countries (*20*). In Bangladesh these accounted for 10–17% of maternal deaths according to community studies (*16, 21*) and 11% of such deaths in Papua New Guinea (*22*). Obstructed labour and its sequelae are the most important causes of maternal death in tropical Africa.

In most cases of obstructed delivery, the problem arises because the space in the bony birth canal of the mother is either too small or too distorted by disease to permit easy passage of the head of the baby during labour. A point of special relevance to any discussion of obstructed labour is that maternal stature and the size of the space in the maternal pelvis are related. The relationship is such that the proportion of women with small pelvises decreases steadily with increasing height, so that difficult labour due to a small pelvis is rare in tall women, and comparatively common in short women. In northern Nigeria, for example, of those mothers having their first babies who received prenatal care, the proportion with a small pelvis who required operative delivery varied from 40% among women under 1.45 metres tall to 14% of those 1.50 metres tall, and to less than 1% of mothers who were 1.60 metres or taller (*23*). Similarly a

---

[1] Mafiamba, P. C. *Problems of human reproduction in Cameroon.* Paper prepared for the WHO Regional Multidisciplinary Consultative Meeting on Human Reproduction, Yaoundé, 4–7 December 1978. Unpublished WHO document HRP/RMC/78.4.

study in the Gambia found that teenage mothers under 1.55 m tall who had babies weighing over 2.95 kg had a forceps delivery rate of 20% and a caesarean section rate of 6.7%, compared with rates of 8.9% and 3.1%, respectively, for taller women of the same age delivering similar-sized babies (24).

Genetic, physiological and environmental factors, including nutrition, all affect the stature of a person. In places where living standards are good and the population is healthy and well fed, most mothers attain their genetically determined maximum stature by the time growth in height ceases at about the age of 18 years. Growth in the bony pelvis stops some three years later (25). Under less favourable conditions, where environmental hygiene is poor and malnutrition and infectious diseases such as malaria, diarrhoea and measles are rife, growth in stature will be slowed, causing stunting.

Mention must also be made of osteomalacia, a disease of bone which affects pelvic size. Calcium and vitamin D are both important in the formation of normal bone. Calcium is obtained from the diet (milk products are rich sources); vitamin D is obtained both from the diet (principally animal products, especially milk and eggs) and from the action of direct sunlight on certain chemical substances in the skin. Vitamin D deficiency, resulting from either dietary inadequacy or lack of exposure to sunlight (as in women in purdah), impairs the deposition of calcium in the bones. Under such circumstances the pelvis may become contracted and may also become deformed in shape. The condition was once common among the poor in large industrial cities of Europe. Nowadays in Europe, osteomalacia continues to be seen among certain sections of the immigrant population (26).

Some of the most extreme forms of pelvic contraction are found in societies where there is mass poverty and where it is customary for childbearing to begin before girls are fully grown. In such areas, for example, northern Nigeria and the Sudan, labour is often obstructed at the time of the birth of the first baby. The principal way to relieve the obstruction and so save the lives of both mother and baby is to perform a caesarean section. If the condition is not dealt with in its early stages, the obstruction can last for days and may result in the death of the mother through infection and exhaustion, and death of the fetus through infection, birth injury and lack of oxygen. If antibiotic treatment is not given, infection sets in within about twelve hours of the membranes rupturing in a high proportion of women with obstructed labour, and in nearly 100% of women who remain undelivered after 24 hours. Sometimes infection is the result of traditional treatment for prolonged labour, such as the administration of herbs or other substances to the vagina (see also Chapter 7).

Not infrequently, women with obstructed labour arrive at hospital with the baby still undelivered but already dead in the womb. Although caesarean section can relieve the obstruction in such cases, a special kind of assisted vaginal delivery is more often used, whereby instruments are passed through the vagina and the dead fetus is cut up or crushed to reduce its bulk before traction is applied to deliver it.

Rupture of the uterus is another major complication of obstructed labour. Extremely rare in women giving birth for the first time, it may be a common occurrence in those who have borne several children. A study in Uganda found an incidence of 11 cases of ruptured uterus per 1000 deliveries (27), compared with 16 per 1000 deliveries in a study from Ghana (28), 2.4 per 1000 in a study from India (29), and 7.4 per 1000 in a study from Honduras (30). Once the uterus ruptures there is severe pain and tenderness over it, heavy bleeding from the torn vessels of the uterus follows and death results from haemorrhage and shock within 24 hours, or from infection later. Surgical treatment, aimed at arresting the bleeding, is always necessary if the mother is to survive. This is achieved either by repairing the tear in the uterus or by removing the uterus (hysterectomy).

The prevention of obstructed labour and its sequelae requires action on both a medical and a sociocultural level. In the latter context, first and foremost is the need to reduce the proportion of women with pelvic contraction in the child-bearing population. Delaying marriage until women have reached full physical maturity is obviously desirable, and one way of achieving this is through compulsory, universal, formal education. In some places, however, such a social policy might come into conflict with deeply rooted traditional customs and would be difficult to introduce. Better nutrition and improvements in living conditions are also important because they help to prevent stunted growth (see also Chapter 4).

As far as the health service is concerned, the role of health personnel is to recognize in good time the expectant mothers who are at risk of obstructed labour, and to ensure they deliver where skilled help is available. Women less than 1.50 metres tall, girls in the early teenage years, and expectant mothers who have had a prolonged labour, instrumental vaginal delivery or abdominal delivery on a previous occasion, are all at risk. For these women, delivery in hospital offers the best prospect. However, under the conditions that prevail in many developing countries, it would be naive to expect all such women to deliver in hospital. Even so, people can be made to understand that prolonged labour is exceedingly dangerous, and that for a woman who has been in labour at home for 24 hours without delivering, immediate transfer to hospital offers the best chance of survival, provided that the hospital is equipped to handle complicated cases (see Chapter 8).

## Haemorrhage

Bleeding related to late pregnancy and delivery can be conveniently considered under two main headings: antepartum haemorrhage, in which vaginal bleeding occurs before the child is born; and postpartum haemorrhage, where excessive bleeding begins shortly after the birth of the baby.

### Antepartum haemorrhage

Episodes of bleeding through the vagina during pregnancy are always abnormal. When such bleeding occurs before the 28th week of pregnancy, it is commonly associated with abortion of one kind or another. Bleeding after the 28th week of pregnancy may be due to premature separation of the placenta, or to injury, or even to disease affecting the lower genital tract, though this last is rare. In cases where the bleeding is associated with placental separation, the eventual outcome will depend partly on the position of the placenta within the uterus. Normally it is attached to the inner surface of the upper part of the uterus, and bleeding associated with a placenta in this position is called accidental haemorrhage. Women aged 35 years or over and those with four or more previous births are more commonly affected than those who are younger or of lower parity. The underprivileged are also more vulnerable to accidental haemorrhage than the well-to-do, though the reason for this difference is not known. In its severe form, accidental haemorrhage produces very acute abdominal pain. This, in conjunction with the bleeding, most of which is concealed within the uterus, quickly produces severe shock in the mother and the death of the baby.

There are additional dangers to maternal life apart from the bleeding. The circulating blood may lose some of its most important qualities, one being the ability to clot normally. The risk of further heavy bleeding then increases markedly. The other danger to maternal life is kidney failure, encountered chiefly where treatment has been unduly delayed. As the kidneys fail, they are no longer able to perform their normal function of ridding the body of its waste products, which accumulate and poison practically all other systems in the body. The condition can be fatal in a matter of days. In most developing countries, the treatment of kidney failure is well beyond the means of the vast majority of hospitals, because of the expense and the technical expertise involved.

Severe accidental haemorrhage is a grave obstetric emergency. The primary objective of treatment is to terminate the pregnancy, but not before measures have been taken to improve the general health of the woman. Such measures include the control of pain by the use of powerful pain-relieving drugs, and the replacement of blood loss by blood transfusion.

Placenta praevia is the other type of antepartum haemorrhage. Here the bleeding is from the separation of a placenta whose position in the uterus is abnormal, in that it is attached partly or entirely to the inner surface of the lower part of the uterus. In the presence of placenta praevia, the baby commonly assumes an abnormal position. It may, for example, be lying with the breech (buttocks) or even the shoulder positioned directly above the low-lying placenta, whereas normally the fetal head occupies the lower pole of the uterus.

There are other characteristics of bleeding in placenta praevia. It is rarely associated with abdominal pain unless the mother happens to be in labour. Typically, the bleeding is very slight at first and it soon stops; other episodes of bleeding follow, and these are all intermittent, unpredictable and of increasing severity.

A pregnant woman suspected of having placenta praevia requires expert supervision. The aim is always to prolong the pregnancy until a mature baby can be born, and in the meantime to take steps to improve the health of the mother. Blood replacement by transfusion may be necessary. It is best to deliver the baby around the 38th week of gestation, and the choice between induction of labour and caesarean section depends on clinical and technical considerations which are beyond the scope of this discussion.

Like accidental haemorrhage, placenta praevia is associated with high parity, and so is more common in places where it is customary to have large families.

## Postpartum haemorrhage

Postpartum haemorrhage refers to excessive bleeding through the birth canal after the birth of the baby. The action of the uterus during labour is directed not only towards expelling the baby and the placenta but also towards closing down the blood vessels afterwards. Normally the placenta is expelled within 30 minutes of the birth of the baby, and uterine contractions continue so that bleeding soon stops. For a variety of reasons the placenta may fail to separate, and bleeding will not stop altogether for as long as the placenta, or part of it, remains in the uterus. Apart from retained placenta, other causes of postpartum haemorrhage include prolonged labour, all forms of operative vaginal delivery, the action of anaesthetic agents, and uterine tumours such as fibroids. Women with a multiple pregnancy and those who have had four or more previous births are particularly at risk of postpartum haemorrhage, probably because the uterine muscles have been overstretched and are less able to contract normally. A study in Papua New Guinea, for example, found that of maternal deaths caused by postpartum haemorrhage, 17% were among women giving birth for the first time, compared with 44% among women who had had four or more previous births (22). Nearly half of the latter were associated with prolonged retention of the placenta.

Heavy bleeding can also result from injuries caused during childbirth, either spontaneously or during operative delivery. Rupture of the uterus, tears in the cervix and vagina, and injuries lower down the birth canal and the perineum can all cause haemorrhage.

## Ectopic pregnancy

Ectopic pregnancy is another important cause of heavy bleeding. In this condition, the implantation of the fertilized ovum and its subsequent development, both of which normally take place in the uterus, occur outside it. The commonest site for an ectopic pregnancy is the fallopian tube. Because it cannot accommodate the growing embryo and fetus, the fallopian tube soon ruptures (usually within the first 10 weeks of pregnancy), there is bleeding and the blood accumulates in the abdomen, producing intense local and generalized pain, fainting and shock. Left untreated, ectopic pregnancy can be fatal in a matter of hours. Surgery is necessary: the abdomen is opened and the affected fallopian tube removed and its blood vessels tied off to stop further bleeding. Replacement of blood loss is almost always required.

An analysis of maternal deaths in Jamaica from 1981 to 1983 (*15*) revealed that ectopic pregnancy was responsible for 10% of such deaths (for further discussion of incidence and causes, see Chapter 7).

## Mortality and treatment

The risk of dying from haemorrhage depends on the amount and rate of blood loss and on the state of health of the patient. A woman with antepartum haemorrhage is estimated to have around 12 hours to live unless she receives treatment, and a woman with postpartum haemorrhage only 2 hours. Any woman who develops obstetric haemorrhage and whose home is remote from medical services is obviously in a perilous position. Not surprisingly, haemorrhage is the biggest single cause of maternal death in many reports from developing countries. In selected community studies it accounted for over 31% of direct obstetric deaths in Fiji (*7*), for 54% in Menoufia, Egypt (*17*), 67% in Bali (*17*), and 33% in Papua New Guinea (*22*).

No matter what the cause of the bleeding, death is always from one or more of the following effects—shock, anaemia, infection, kidney failure or brain damage. Sometimes death occurs long after the obstetric condition initially responsible for the haemorrhage has ceased to exist.

Prenatal care has an important role to play in preventing deaths from haemorrhage by identifying early in pregnancy those women who are at particular risk, and encouraging them to deliver in hospital.

## Anaemia

Anaemia is the term used to describe the condition in which there is a reduction of the concentration of haemoglobin in the bloodstream to a level (for pregnant women) below

110 g/l (*31*).[1] Haemoglobin is the red pigment present in solution in the red corpuscles of the blood, and its primary function is to transport oxygen to all parts of the body. Iron, folic acid, other vitamins, and trace elements are all required for the formation of haemoglobin, which takes place in the bone marrow. These substances are all ingested from food; green vegetables and such staples as potatoes and yams are important sources of folic acid, and most cereals, meat and vegetables contain iron.

Under normal circumstances not all the iron ingested and absorbed daily from the small intestine is needed immediately. The excess is usually stored in the bone marrow, so that during periods of physical stress it can be used to increase the rate of formation of haemoglobin to satisfy increased needs. One such period of physical stress is pregnancy.

During pregnancy, growth of the fetus and of the uterus, and other changes taking place in the expectant mother, lead to an increase in the demand for many nutrients, especially iron and folic acid. Since most women in the Third World start pregnancy with depleted body stores of these nutrients, their extra requirement is even higher than usual. If, because of dietary deficiencies, these needs are not met, the rate of formation of haemoglobin declines and its concentration in the circulating blood falls.

Apart from nutritional deficiency of iron and folic acid, there are other causes of anaemia. Malaria, sickle cell disease, bacterial infections, and blood loss from abortion, ectopic pregnancy or intestinal parasites such as hookworms are all important causes. In malaria and sickle cell disease, red blood corpuscles are destroyed faster than the body can replace them. In the case of bacterial infections, normal bone marrow function is suppressed so that even if the relevant nutrients are all present in the body their conversion to haemoglobin cannot take place until the infection is brought under control. In the course of blood loss from the causes mentioned above, red corpuscles, and hence haemoglobin, are lost. If the haemorrhage is very heavy, the haemoglobin concentration will fall and will remain low until the lost red cells are replaced.

---

[1] This is the level recommended by a WHO Expert Committee. Some obstetricians in developing countries feel that 100 g/l would be more appropriate.

Behind the medical causes of anaemia, socioeconomic factors play an important role. The extent of poverty in developing countries largely explains why severe anaemia is so common and why its effects are so serious throughout most of the Third World. About two-thirds of pregnant women in developing countries (excluding China) are estimated to be anaemic (*32*), compared with 14% in developed countries (*33*). Hardships imposed by poor nutrition, water shortage, food taboos, inadequacies in food production and storage, and absence of effective systems of social security all combine to undermine women's health and cause anaemia as well as a host of other debilitating diseases.

The early stages of anaemia in pregnancy are often without symptoms. However, as the haemoglobin concentration falls, oxygen supply to vital organs declines, and the expectant mother begins to complain of general weakness, tiredness, dizziness, and headaches. Pallor of the skin and of the mucous membranes, as well as the nail beds and tongue, becomes noticeable when the haemoglobin drops to 70 g/l. With a further fall in haemoglobin concentration to 40 g/l, most tissues of the body become starved of oxygen, and the effect is most marked on the heart muscles, which may fail altogether if there is severe anaemia. Death from anaemia is the result of heart failure, shock, or infection that has taken advantage of the patient's impaired resistance to disease. Anaemia was the primary cause of an upsurge in maternal deaths among women in two refugee camps in Somalia in 1987 (B. Farah et al., unpublished data). Of the 44 deaths recorded, 42 were associated with anaemia. Although many of the women were first noted to be severely anaemic in the third trimester of pregnancy, severe anaemia was not noted in some until after delivery and often only after several weeks of diarrhoea and vomiting or other illness. Fortunately the extreme deprivation suffered by such refugee women is not common, but even in Fiji, for example, anaemia was given as the direct cause of between 4% and 12% of all maternal deaths between 1969 and 1976 (*7*).

However, figures such as these do not tell the whole story. While less severe anaemia may not be a direct cause of maternal death, it can contribute towards death from other causes. Anaemic mothers do not tolerate blood loss to the same extent as healthy women. During childbirth, blood loss of up to one litre will not kill a healthy woman, but in a grossly anaemic woman, a loss of as little as 150 ml can be fatal. Anaemic women are poor anaesthetic and operative risks. As already stated, anaemia lowers resistance to infection and for this reason, after surgery, wounds may fail to heal promptly or may break down altogether. In Papua New Guinea the higher rate of death from obstetric haemorrhage reported in the coastal region as compared with the highlands is thought to be associated with higher rates of anaemia at the coast (22). And a review of the symptoms associated with maternal deaths in a study in Tangail, Bangladesh, led researchers to conclude that anaemia had played a secondary role in nearly every case (21).

Tests on the blood, urine and faeces are often sufficient to establish the cause of anaemia and thus the correct form of treatment. Most of these tests are within the means of hospitals in developing countries. Treatment of anaemia in pregnancy often involves supplementary iron and folic acid coupled with malaria chemoprophylaxis in places where malaria is endemic. The latter is important because the immunity to malaria built up during repeated attacks in childhood begins to break down in pregnant women at about the 14th week, for reasons that are not yet known. The process is most marked in first pregnancies. A well balanced diet also helps to correct anaemia.

Treatment along these lines takes four weeks or longer to restore the haemoglobin concentration to something like the normal level. Thus the real problem arises when severe anaemia is seen for the first time towards the end of pregnancy, or during abortion or in labour, because on these occasions there is not enough time for treatment with iron, folic acid and antimalarial drugs to correct the condition before the patient aborts or delivers. Under such circumstances, the bleeding that normally follows abortion or delivery can be fatal. The only way in which the low haemoglobin concentration can be raised quickly to a safe level is through blood transfusion.

Iron and folic acid supplements, together with malarial chemoprophylaxis taken throughout pregnancy, have long been known to prevent severe anaemia in most areas in the Third World. In addition, screening for anaemia three times during pregnancy—at the first visit for prenatal care, at the 30th week and at the 36th week—is always worth while. In this way, it should be possible to identify those who fail to comply with treatment, and others who are anaemic for other reasons, such as sickle cell disease.

Another important point is that anaemic women who have a low erythrocyte volume fraction (haematocrit) are much more likely to die than women with normal levels. (This is the ratio of volume of red cells to the volume of whole blood, and it is measured by centrifuging a sample of blood to separate out the components.) However, a very high erythrocyte volume fraction in a pregnant woman can be dangerous too in that it may indicate a change in the composition of the blood whereby the fluid is reduced in amount but not the red blood cells. Women with eclampsia, ruptured uterus, and untreated obstructed labour are particularly prone to become short of body fluids to the extent that it affects the composition of their blood. When such women then lose blood during delivery or operation, replacement of the loss by blood transfusion may be dangerous. In a study in Zaria, Nigeria (*34*), as many as one-third of those treated in this way died compared with 1 in 10 of those who were not given a blood transfusion. For such women, replacement of the fluid loss by glucose solution appears to be a safer course of action. This finding has important implications for reducing maternal mortality. More lives could be saved if the erythrocyte volume fraction towards the end of pregnancy, and better still during labour, were known in women with major obstetric complications.

## Puerperal (or genital) sepsis

For various reasons, women are particularly prone to infection of the genital tract following delivery and abortion. The site in the uterus at which the placenta was attached is left as a raw area until it is covered by a fresh lining of cells within a few weeks. Tears in the lining of the genital tract occur as a result of the birth, leaving some of the tissues bruised and without proper blood supply. In the first few days following childbirth or abortion, the vulva, vagina and cervix are all open in a way that they are not at any other time in a woman's life. In addition, blood clots, tissue fragments, and pieces of the products of conception abound, and these may become infected.

The offending germs may enter the genital tract in various ways, e.g., if the birth attendant has unclean hands or uses dirty instruments. Infection can also be conveyed from dust in the atmosphere, or the mother herself can start the process by the transfer of infective organisms from various sites, especially the anus. The insertion of foreign objects into the vagina during labour, such as herbs, leaves, cow dung, mud, or various oils, by traditional attendants is also a cause of infection (see also Chapter 7).

Puerperal infection following a straightforward spontaneous normal delivery is extremely rare, no matter how unhygienic the surroundings, provided that nothing is introduced into the vagina during labour. However, many women in the Third World do not have straightforward deliveries, and are subject to harmful interference during labour by untrained attendants who do not appreciate the significance of hygiene. As a result, puerperal sepsis is one of the three most important causes of maternal death in developing countries, and rates are particularly high where there are also high rates of illicit abortion (see also Chapter 6).

For example, a study of maternal mortality in 1982–83 in Jamalpur, Bangladesh (16) found that 31% of all maternal deaths were due to infection, 21% of which followed abortion. In a report from the southern highlands of the United Republic of Tanzania, 37 of the 115 maternal deaths were due to infection (35). Twenty of these deaths were associated with abortion, and the author suggests that the habit of inserting cloths into the vagina after delivery to soak up the discharge also played a part.

When it starts, infection is generally confined to the uterus; at this stage there is some pain and tenderness in the lower abdomen, with an offensive vaginal discharge. Fever, increasing abdominal pain, vomiting, headache, and loss of appetite indicate the spread of the infection to other sites. Abscesses may form within the fallopian tubes, the pelvis, and underneath the diaphragm. In severe cases, the infection can spread into the bloodstream (septicaemia), giving rise to abscesses in the brain, muscles and kidneys. If the infection is not controlled, mental disorientation and coma set in and death occurs from a wide variety of complications, including shock, kidney failure, liver failure and anaemia. Sepsis is fatal within about six days of the onset if no treatment is given.

Treatment is straightforward in early cases, but complicated in advanced disease. When puerperal sepsis is mild, and the infecting organism is still confined to the uterus and genital tract, measures to improve the general health, such as a balanced diet, rest and the use of drugs to relieve the pain, will enable the body to fight the germs. Once the spread of the germs has been checked, the affected mother often recovers within about two weeks.

Antibiotics also play an important part in the treatment of puerperal sepsis. Nowadays, there are many of these drugs to choose from and in theory they should always succeed in curing puerperal sepsis. But in practice the outlook is not so good. The germs that cause puerperal sepsis are becoming increasingly resistant to antibiotics, largely as a result of the indiscriminate use of the drugs. If a patient fails to complete a course of treatment with antibiotics, stopping as soon as the symptoms are relieved, the remaining organisms can once again start to multiply, producing a strain that is more resistant to the antibiotic.

Any abscesses need to be drained, and some patients with extensive disease may need to undergo hysterectomy.

Of measures to reduce deaths from puerperal infection, cleanliness and asepsis during labour are of prime importance. It is best to avoid vaginal examination altogether in circumstances where standards of asepsis and antisepsis are suspect. On a wider scale, communities themselves have an important part to play in reducing the incidence of puerperal infection, and health workers particularly should remind those in positions of power and authority that the control of bacterial infection improves when water for washing becomes freely available and when soap is sold at prices that everyone can afford. In short, improvements in personal and environmental hygiene, both within and outside hospital, are very important in the control of puerperal sepsis.

## Jaundice in pregnancy and acute liver failure

Malaria, certain blood diseases and hepatitis can cause jaundice and threaten life during pregnancy. The present discussion will be confined to viral hepatitis, a disease in which the liver is invaded and injured by certain viruses and to which pregnant women seem to be especially susceptible. Studies from Ethiopia and the Islamic Republic of Iran, for example, show that the incidence of viral hepatitis for pregnant women is twice as high as for non-pregnant women and that pregnant women are more seriously ill and are more likely to die. Case–fatality rates are up to 3.5 times higher than in non-pregnant women (36–38). In Addis Ababa in 1983, viral hepatitis was the third largest cause of maternal death (39).

There are three forms of viral hepatitis: hepatitis A, hepatitis B, and hepatitis non-A, non-B. The virus that causes hepatitis A is excreted in human faeces; therefore an important cause of disease is the faecal contamination of food and drinking-water. For example, consumption of raw or inadequately cooked shellfish grown in faecally contaminated shallow water, of raw vegetables grown in fields fertilized with untreated human faeces, and of drinking-water from open drains and from shallow wells unprotected against faecal contamination all greatly increase the risk of infection with hepatitis A virus.

The virus that causes hepatitis B is carried in body fluids such as blood, saliva, semen and vaginal secretions, and is transmitted through close bodily contact. Infected blood is an important source of this disease, and health workers handling blood are particularly vulnerable.

There are at least two agents that cause non-A non-B hepatitis and transmission may be by the faecal–oral route or through close bodily contact.

In viral hepatitis, the extent of the injury to the liver varies. Where damage is mild, the liver cells that are unaffected rapidly multiply to replace those that are injured. In this way, normal liver function is maintained and the patient recovers. Less commonly, the liver may be destroyed entirely, making regeneration impossible and death of the patient inevitable.

Reports from Africa (*10, 40*) and the eastern Mediterranean area (*6*) reveal that women of low socioeconomic status in these areas are particularly susceptible to viral hepatitis, and that the agents mostly responsible for the disease in pregnant women are hepatitis A and non-A non-B hepatitis viruses. Early symptoms of viral hepatitis are general weakness, increasing tiredness, fever, headache and joint pains. Loss of appetite, nausea, vomiting, pain in the upper abdomen and finally jaundice follow. The jaundice may deepen rapidly and in mild cases fades as the affected mother slowly recovers.

Viral hepatitis in its fulminating form occurs most often in the third trimester of pregnancy. Premature labour, liver failure and severe haemorrhage commonly complicate this form of the disease, and many infants are born too soon to survive. The mothers who die do so from liver failure and from severe haemorrhage. Fatal haemorrhage in these cases is triggered by acute liver failure. In this condition the blood loses its ability to clot, and bleeding occurs not only through the birth canal but also into other sites such as the stomach, intestines, mucous membranes and injection sites in the skin and muscle.

Treatment of viral hepatitis involves complete bed rest and a special diet to reduce the work of the liver until it can recover its function. Good sanitation greatly reduces the risk of viral hepatitis.

## Operative deliveries

In most large hospitals in developing countries about 85% of deliveries are normal. The rest are operative deliveries and they take several forms. In some, the manipulations needed to extract the baby are carried out vaginally. Obstetric forceps, vacuum extraction and destruction of the fetus are examples of operative vaginal delivery. The other group of operative deliveries is abdominal, caesarean section being the commonest.

As may be expected, normal spontaneous vaginal delivery is by far the safest. Death from complications in the puerperium following normal delivery is possible but rare, particularly in mothers who were free from disease during pregnancy.

In contrast, all operative deliveries carry risks to the mother and infant. The risks arise partly from the nature of the operations, partly from other procedures that go hand in hand with operative deliveries, such as anaesthesia and blood transfusion, and partly from the pregnancy complication which necessitated the operation in the first place. In addition, complications may develop after operative delivery, including severe bleeding and infection. Much will depend on the quality of care available.

Destructive operations carried out in patients admitted as emergencies are particularly risky, not so much because of the technical difficulties of the procedure but because the women who need these operations are, without exception, extremely ill, many having been in advanced obstructed labour for days at home before they arrive in hospital.

## Other medical causes of maternal deaths

Embolism, sickle cell disease and complications associated with anaesthesia currently contribute little towards the high death rate during pregnancy in the Third World, since their effects are overshadowed by those of the major causes of maternal mortality. However, improvements in living conditions and in basic health care services will eventually result in a fall in the number of deaths from haemorrhage, abortion, anaemia, obstructed labour, puerperal sepsis and hypertensive diseases of pregnancy. At that time, deaths due to embolism, sickle cell disease and anaesthetic mishaps will assume greater importance, and so they merit brief discussion here.

An embolus is a plug of material, such as fat, amniotic fluid, air or blood clot, that blocks a blood vessel. In pregnant women, emboli formed from blood clot are the commonest variety. Typically, the clot starts to form in the veins of the lower limbs and the pelvis. From these primary sites, fragments become detached and enter the general circulation, and may eventually become lodged in the lungs. Women over the age of 35 years, those who are overweight and those whose child was delivered by caesarean section are especially at risk. Although the disease may occur during pregnancy, especially in women with varicose veins, it is commonest between the 5th and the 15th day after delivery. Warning signs of embolism are usually slight. Low-grade fever and pain in the calf muscles are ominous, but pulmonary embolism becomes obvious when sudden chest pain, acute breathlessness and collapse occur. Treatment involves the use of anticoagulant drugs and intensive care of a kind that most developing countries cannot afford.

Air embolism is associated with illegal abortion, while fat emboli occur in women with sickle cell disease. Black Africans and their descendants are chiefly affected by sickle cell disease. The term sickle cell disease is used to describe a group of inherited blood diseases in which there is an abnormality in the chemical structure of the haemoglobin. This chemical abnormality alters the character of the red corpuscles, which contain the haemoglobin. The affected red cells are more easily destroyed, leading to anaemia. The other feature of sickle cell disease is intermittent, severe pain in the bones and other organs of the body. The reason for this is fairly straightforward. In sickle cell disease the membrane that covers the red corpuscles sometimes becomes rigid and misshapen. This hinders the free passage of the red cells through the smallest blood vessels. Blockage of the small vessels impedes blood flow so that the affected tissues are starved of oxygen and nutrients and severe pain and tenderness develop over them.

In expectant mothers with sickle cell disease, the last four weeks of pregnancy, labour and the first week after delivery are particularly dangerous, and most of the maternal deaths occur during this period. Deaths result from the effects of embolism, anaemia, and bacterial infections. Treatment during pregnancy involves the prevention of anaemia and the control of infection.

Improvements in anaesthetic techniques and technical expertise are among the most important reasons for the fall in the maternal mortality rate in developed countries. The anaesthetic technique used must not only relieve pain; it must also keep the patient's airway open because at all times oxygen must be able to pass freely through the respiratory passages into the bloodstream. Difficulties arise when the airway is blocked. Sometimes tubes meant to keep the airway open are wrongly positioned, or may become blocked when a patient vomits and inhales the stomach contents. Failure to recognize these accidents early leads rapidly to death from cardiac and respiratory arrest and sometimes from gas embolism.

## Regional variations and changes over time in the main causes of death

The types of pregnancy complications seen in countries where maternal mortality rates are high are remarkably similar. While certain causes of death, such as viral hepatitis and tetanus, are significant in some areas of the world but not in others, haemorrhage, sepsis and toxaemia are important everywhere.

Most of the information on causes of maternal death comes from hospitals; Table 5.1 (page 76) summarized hospital reports from Africa, Asia, Latin America and the Pacific. In Africa, obstructed labour with uterine rupture, hypertensive disease of pregnancy, sepsis and haemorrhage are undoubtedly the main problems. In Asia, the problems are similar but severe anaemia also plays a very important part. And in Latin America, abortion is particularly important as a cause of death.

Community studies, where they exist, show similar patterns (see Table 5.2) but the order of importance of each type of cause can be very different from those seen in hospital, especially where hospital delivery is unusual. This is well illustrated by a study carried out in Jamalpur, Bangladesh where, of 58 deaths, only three occurred in hospital. These

95

Table 5.2. Main causes of maternal death in community studies in developing countries (as percentage of all direct obstetric causes)

| Area | Haemorrhage % | Sepsis % | Toxaemia % | Abortion % | Obstructed labour/ ruptured uterus % | Source (reference) |
|---|---|---|---|---|---|---|
| **Bangladesh** | | | | | | |
| Matlab | 22 | 3 | 19 | 31 | 9 | a |
| Tangail | 17 | 10 | 15 | 10 | 21 | 21 |
| Jamalpur | 12 | 12 | 24 | 24 | 20 | 16 |
| **Colombia** | | | | | | |
| Cali | 22 | – | 34 | 39 | – | b |
| **Cuba** | 6 | 19 | 12 | 15 | – | 41 |
| **Egypt** | | | | | | |
| Menoufia | 54 | 18 | 10 | 7 | – | 17 |
| Upper Egypt | 38 | 11 | 18 | 4 | 8 | c |
| **Ethiopia** | | | | | | |
| Addis Ababa | 12 | 4 | 12 | 54 | 8 | 39 |
| **Indonesia** | | | | | | |
| Bali | 67 | 8 | 7 | 10 | – | 23 |
| **Jamaica** | 23 | 9 | 30 | 6 | 3 | 15 |
| **Papua New Guinea** | 33 | 31 | 4 | 5 | 11 | 22 |

a Lindpainter, L. S. et al. *Maternal mortality in Matlab thana, Bangladesh, 1982.* Unpublished document of the International Centre for Diarrhoeal Diseases Research, Dhaka, Bangladesh.
b Rodriguez, J. et al. Avoidable mortality and maternal mortality in Cali, Colombia. In: *Interregional Meeting on the Prevention of Maternal Mortality. Geneva 11–15 November 1985.* Unpublished WHO document FHE/PMM/85.9.1.
c Abdullah, S. A. et al. Maternal mortality in Upper Egypt. In: *Interregional Meeting on the Prevention of Maternal Mortality. Geneva, 11–15 November 1985.* Unpublished WHO document, FHE/PMM/85.9.18.

three were due to toxaemia, which thus accounted for 100% of hospital deaths, whereas it accounted for only 20% of all the maternal deaths (*16*) (see Table 5.3).

Table 5.3.   Number of maternal deaths, by place and cause of death, in Jamalpur study

| Cause of death | Number of maternal deaths | | | | | |
|---|---|---|---|---|---|---|
| | In own home | In parents' home | In hospital | In *thana* health centre | Other | Total |
| Infection[a] | 15 | 6 | 0 | 1 | 0 | 22 |
| Toxaemia | 7 | 2 | 3 | 0 | 0 | 12 |
| Haemorrhage | 6 | 0 | 0 | 0 | 0. | 6 |
| Difficult labour | 8 | 1 | 0 | 0 | 1 | 10 |
| Other | 8 | 0 | 0 | 0 | 0 | 8 |
| Total | 44 | 9 | 3 | 1 | 1 | 58 |

[a] Includes tetanus, septic abortion, and postpartum sepsis.

*Source*: Khan et al. (*16*).

## Evolution of causes

As countries make progress in bringing down the levels of maternal mortality, the changes in the relative importance of each of the main causes of death can be instructive.

In Cuba, where maternal and child health care has been one of the priorities since the National Health Service was started in 1961, maternal mortality dropped by 73% between 1962 and 1984—from 118 to 31 per 100 000 live births. The most dramatic declines have been seen in deaths from toxaemia and haemorrhage (see Table 5.4).

Table 5.4.   Direct maternal deaths by cause (per 100 000 live births) in Cuba

| Cause | 1960 | 1970 | 1975 | 1980 | 1984 |
|---|---|---|---|---|---|
| Toxaemia | 35 | 6 | 11 | 4 | 4 |
| Haemorrhage | 32 | 8 | 6 | 6 | 2 |
| Abortion | 14 | 22 | 12 | 15 | 5 |
| Sepsis (postpartum) | 9 | 8 | 12 | 9 | 6 |
| Other | 29 | 28 | 27 | 19 | 15 |
| All direct causes | 119 | 72 | 68 | 53 | 32 |

*Source*: Farnot Cardoso (*41*).

Since 1961 extra hospitals have been built in the previously underserved rural areas of Cuba; prenatal care has become widely available, and "maternity waiting homes" have been established so that women from remote areas who are at risk of suffering complications in labour can move near to hospital towards the end of their pregnancies. By 1984 delivery in health institutions had increased to 99% from a level of 63% in 1963. It seems likely, therefore, that the reduction in mortality from toxaemia and haemorrhage can in large part be attributed to the spread of better health care offering regular surveillance and speedy treatment for these conditions.

This appears to have been the case also in Jamaica, where a marked decline in maternal mortality (from 373 in 1950–52 to 48 per 100 000 live births in 1977–79, according to civil registration data) was also the result of increasing commitment to maternal health care and hospital delivery (31). Here the absolute number of deaths from toxaemia fell from 186 to 28 in the same period, and deaths from haemorrhage fell from 84 to 13.

The proportional decline in the different causes depends to a large extent on the overall level of maternal mortality. Haemorrhage and sepsis are usually the most important causes where overall levels of maternal mortality are high. As levels decline the relative importance of these two causes diminishes and other causes such as toxaemia become more important. In Cuba between 1960 and 1984, for instance, there was only a small reduction in mortality from infection, because the overall level of maternal mortality was already relatively low at the beginning of this period. Data from Sri Lanka on the other hand show how, during a decline from very high levels, sepsis declined first, accounting for about 25% of maternal deaths in 1950–55 to 3% in 1979, excluding abortion (see Fig. 5.1).[1] In China, too, where the overall maternal mortality rate in Beijing, for example, has fallen from 685 per 100 000 live births in 1949 to 23 per 100 000 in 1983 (42), a survey carried out in 21 provinces showed that sepsis now accounts for only about 6% of deaths (43).

A decline in the number of deaths from sepsis generally reflects better standards of hygiene (such as the emphasis on

___

[1] Vidyasagara, N. W. *Maternal services in Sri Lanka*. Unpublished paper presented at the tenth Asian and Oceanic Congress of Obstetrics and Gynaecology, Colombo, 4–10 September 1985.

Fig. 5.1. Trends in certain causes of maternal mortality, Sri Lanka, 1953–1968

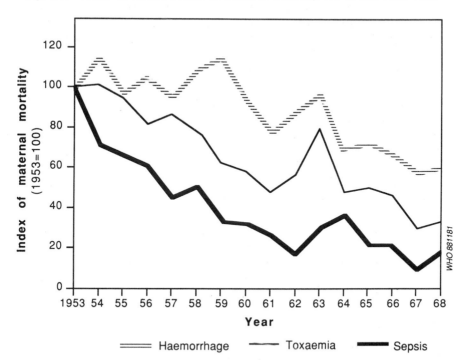

Note. Figures are cause-specific maternal mortality rates expressed as a percentage of the rates in 1953

the "three cleans" in China: clean hands, clean perineum, clean cord care) and the wider use of antibiotic treatment. This can be accomplished in practically any setting. However, reduction in mortality from haemorrhage requires relatively sophisticated facilities—and, with this cause particularly, there is also a pressing need for speed because of the short time between the onset of serious bleeding and death. This is well demonstrated by the fact that in the rural areas of China, haemorrhage is the leading cause of maternal death, responsible for over 50%, whereas it accounts for only 25% of maternal deaths in urban areas, where hospitals are more readily accessible (43).

## The wider picture of maternal death

In the complex chain of events leading to maternal death, there are some practical considerations that deserve particular mention. These relate to the accessibility and the quality of professional care.

## Logistic problems

A striking feature of maternal mortality in many developing countries is that a considerable majority of the women who die come from rural areas, to an extent quite out of proportion to the rural/urban distribution of the population in question.

This underlines the point that women in remote areas have great difficulty getting to hospital, either in an emergency or for a routine delivery. Often the roads are rough, and may be impassable at certain times of the year; there may be no transport, or a lack of spare parts or fuel to keep vehicles in service. Or people may simply be too poor to afford the fares. Communications may also be disrupted by wars or civil strife.

In many places such problems of access are compounded by the fact that health services are unduly concentrated in urban areas. For example, of 200 obstetricians working in Nigeria in the early 1980s, more than 90% were situated in national and state capitals. A study of maternal mortality in the Farafeni area of the Gambia in 1982–83 found that, while there were fortnightly mother and child health clinics within about 20 km of village women, those needing hospital treatment faced a 200-km journey by ferry to the capital, Banjul (*44*).

It has been estimated that roughly 15–20% of pregnant women will suffer serious complications, so the odds are heavy against those who live in remote communities.

It is also true that women from country villages, unused to a city environment, sometimes complain that they are made to look stupid by some hospital staff. Such women may subsequently avoid hospitals and health professionals at all costs. Thus, psychological barriers to care can be as much of a problem as material ones.

## The quality of care

Very frequently, women who have travelled from afar reach hospital in a desperately sick state, perhaps too late for effective treatment. But delay on the road may not be the only obstacle to survival. In studies from Colombia, India, the United Republic of Tanzania, and Viet Nam, action by health staff in treating patients was identified as a contributory factor in 11–47% of maternal deaths.[1] Another study from the United Republic of Tanzania (35) estimated that about 10% of the maternal deaths under review were caused by failures in the health service (see Tables 5.5 and 5.6), chief among them being lack of blood or equipment to

Table 5.5. Number of deaths in hospital with an avoidable factor, United Republic of Tanzania (series of 89 maternal deaths)

| Main avoidable factor | No. of deaths | Percentage of total |
|---|---|---|
| Lack of blood | 17 | 19.1 |
| No partogram in labour | 16 | 18.0 |
| Risk factor noted but not acted upon | 30 | 33.7 |
| No anti-gas-gangrene serum | 1 | 1.1 |
| No intravenous equipment | 1 | 1.1 |
| "Slow" laboratory | 3 | 3.4 |
| Staff factors | 9 | 10.1 |
| Untreated anaemia | 4 | 4.5 |
| Uncontrolled eclampsia | 3 | 3.4 |
| Untreated asthma | 2 | 2.2 |
| No anticoagulation | 1 | 1.1 |
| Local herbs given | 2 | 2.2 |

*Source*: Price (35).

Table 5.6. Number of deaths outside hospital with an avoidable factor, United Republic of Tanzania (series of 26 maternal deaths)

| Main avoidable factor | No. of deaths | Percentage of total |
|---|---|---|
| Risk factor not acted upon after detection: | | |
| in village | 10 | 38.5 |
| at health centre | 4 | 15.4 |
| at dispensary | 3 | 11.5 |
| Delay in referral | 3 | 11.5 |
| Refused admission | 1 | 3.8 |
| Absconded | 1 | 3.8 |
| No transport | 1 | 3.8 |
| Induced abortion | 3 | 11.5 |

*Source*: Price (35).

---

[1] *Prevention of maternal mortality. Report of a WHO Inter-regional Meeting, Geneva, 11–15 November 1985.* Unpublished WHO document FHE/86.1.

carry out transfusions. There was also a lack of appropriate drugs for the treatment of infections, and in several cases staff had failed to take the necessary steps to prevent eclamptic fits, even though signs of the condition had been recognized. Similarly a study from Papua New Guinea (22) revealed that 20% of maternal deaths due to haemorrhage had occurred in health centres. And in Jamaica an inquiry into all maternal deaths occurring between 1981 and 1984 concluded that one or more avoidable factors were present in 68% of the deaths, with the health staff alone carrying responsibility for 58% of these factors (15). They included deficiencies in prenatal care, delays in starting treatment in the presence of eclampsia or pre-eclampsia, misdiagnosis of ectopic pregnancy, as well as non-availability of blood for transfusion.

Such reports are not uncommon: in developing countries resources are limited, needs are very great, and health staff are often overwhelmed by the workload.

## The road to maternal death

The range of problems suggested briefly here and the ways in which they interact with each other to undermine the survival chances of pregnant women in difficulties are perhaps best illustrated by specific case histories. The following were recorded by a team investigating maternal deaths in Addis Ababa.[1]

> Tadelech lived in a remote village high up among rugged mountains and about 160 km from the capital city. The journey from village to city can take days, depending on whether it is undertaken on foot, by mule and later by tractor, by bus or by ambulance.

> Tadelech was 25 years old and had already delivered two children safely in the village. This was her third pregnancy and since she lived too far from even a health station, she had no prenatal care. Contractions started when Tadelech was nine months pregnant. After two days of labour she had severe backache and abdominal pain but delivery was not near. She was carried on a homemade stretcher to a health station where the health assistant referred her to the nearest health centre. There was nothing the nurse at the centre could do to help

---

[1] Kwast, B. E. *Roads to maternal death. Case histories, including comments on preventive strategies.* Informal Paper No. 1. International Safe Motherhood Conference, Nairobi, 1987.

because labour was obstructed. Tadelech's records mention that the baby was dead and that she was bleeding vaginally, which suggested a low lying placenta.

She was transferred to the district hospital. On arrival there she was given an intravenous infusion and the diagnosis of placenta praevia was reiterated. Even though the district hospital was staffed by two doctors, facilities for emergency obstetric operations were not available. This meant another journey of 120 km to the nearest city hospital with operative facilities. The district hospital had an ambulance but the budget for petrol did not include patient referral. The ambulance could be used if the family paid $47. With an average per capita income of $141 per annum, this amount was prohibitive. The family could not pay, so Tadelech spent another 24 hours travelling.

She arrived at the city hospital anaemic and in shock after two days of vaginal bleeding. Treatment was given according to the original diagnosis of antepartum haemorrhage; this was resuscitation with intravenous fluids. Blood for transfusion was not available.

Tadelech's condition deteriorated. Close questioning of the family about the history of labour led the consultant to change the diagnosis to rupture of the uterus. Exploratory surgery ten hours after admission confirmed this diagnosis and a hysterectomy was performed. Tadelech received her first unit of blood during this operation. She died five hours after surgery, and the same long, expensive journey had to be repeated to return the deceased mother to her family for burial.

Balaynesh's death, identified during the community survey, was the reason for our home visit one year after the event. The house was in a quiet corner of the area. The baby had survived and was well. There was one other child, three years of age. The children were taken care of by relatives elsewhere during the day while the father worked. Since there was only one room, our conversation with the father took place in the street. We knew that Balaynesh had prenatal care in the hospital where she also delivered without problems. She was discharged six hours after delivery as was the routine, but she died three weeks later.

The husband was tense, almost hostile, when he related that his wife had fever and convulsions which started several days after delivery. He said that Balaynesh had experienced such fits one other time before this pregnancy, but that they had subsided without treatment. He had taken her to the holy waters for healing, but without success. Holy waters are springs which bubble out of mountain walls at sites of a monk's vision of a saint's good work.

The question why he had not taken Balaynesh back to the hospital for treatment set the husband off on a desperate tirade. The truth was that he had paid $ 90 for her stay in hospital, which should not have exceeded $ 15 for a normal delivery. The watchman had to be given a considerable tip before Balaynesh could be admitted to the hospital, explained her husband. He could not take her back for treatment since he could not borrow any more money.

Balaynesh's death was never explained and it went unrecorded: mother and baby had been entered as living in the hospital statistics. All the anguish and tragedy occurred outside the hospital walls.

## Conclusion

These tragic case histories bear witness to the fact that the death of a woman in pregnancy or childbirth is rarely the result of clinical complications alone. Once complications arise swift access to good quality professional treatment is essential if lives are to be saved. But there is much that needs to be done to prevent the complications in the first place, and for this we have to look beyond the health services, into the lives of the women themselves and the social, economic and cultural environment in which they live.

## References

1. BHASKER RAO, K. Maternal mortality in a teaching hospital in southern India. A 13-year study. *Obstetrics and gynaecology*, **46**(4): 397–400 (1975).
2. JANJUA, S. National mortality in major city hospitals of Pakistan. *Journal of Pakistan Medical Association*, **29**(2): 31–35 (1979).
3. MARZUKI, A. & THAMBU, J. A. Maternal mortality in the government hospitals, West Malaysia 1967–1969. *Medical journal of Malaysia*, **27**(3): 203–206 (1973).
4. VENNEMA, A. Perinatal mortality and maternal mortality at the Provincial Hospital, Quang Ngai, South Vietnam, 1967–1970. *Tropical and geographic medicine*, **27**: 34–38 (1975).
5. CHI, I. C. ET AL. Maternal mortality at twelve teaching hospitals in Indonesia: an epidemiologic analysis. *International journal of gynaecology and obstetrics*, **19**(4): 259–266 (1981).
6. BORAZJANI, G. ET AL. Maternal mortality in South Iran: a seven year survey. *International journal of gynaecology and obstetrics*, **16**(1): 65–69 (1979).
7. BAVADRA, T. V. ET AL. Maternal mortality in Fiji 1969–1976. *Fiji medical journal*, **6**(1): 4–11 (1978).
8. CAFFREY, K. Y. Maternal mortality: a continuing challenge in

tropical practice. A report from Kaduna, northern Nigeria. *East African medical journal*, **56**(6): 274–277 (1979).

9. WABOSO, M. F. The causes of maternal mortality in the eastern states of Nigeria. *Nigerian medical journal*, **3**(2): 99 (1973).

10. AMPOFO, D. A. Causes of maternal death and comments: maternity hospital, Accra 1963–67. *West African medical journal*, **18**(3): 75–81 (1969).

11. BULLOUGH, C. Analysis of maternal deaths in the Central Region of Malawi. *East African medical journal*, **58**(1): 25–36 (1981).

12. MACPHERSON, T. A. A retrospective study of maternal deaths in the Zimbabwean black. *Central African journal of medicine*, **27**(4): 57–60 (1981).

13. MAKOKHA, A. E. Maternal mortality—Kenyatta National Hospital, 1972–1977. *East African medical journal*, **57**(7): 451–460 (1980).

14. MTIMAVALYE, L. A. ET AL. Maternal mortality in Dar es Salaam, Tanzania 1974–1977. *East African medical journal*, **57**(2): 111–118 (1980).

15. WALKER, G. J. ET AL. Maternal mortality in Jamaica. *Lancet*, **1**(8479): 486–488 (1986).

16. KHAN, A. R. ET AL. Maternal mortality in rural Bangladesh. The Jamalpur district. *Studies in family planning*, **17**(1): 7–12 (1986).

17. FORTNEY, J. A. ET AL. *Causes of death to women of reproductive age in Egypt.* East Lansing, Michigan State University, 1984.

18. HOGBERG, U. *Maternal mortality in Sweden.* Umea, Sweden, Umea University, 1985.

19. FAMILY HEALTH INTERNATIONAL. Successful TBA project in Brazil improves health care inexpensively, *Network*, **4**(4): 1–2 (1983).

20. BERNARD, R. P. & SASTRAWINATA, S. Maternal and perinatal death in Indonesia University obstetrics. Risk display for selected social and biological determinants. In: Lasser, R. et al., ed. *Primary health care in the making*. Heidelberg & Berlin (West), Springer, 1985.

21. ALAUDDIN, M. Maternal mortality in rural Bangladesh. The Tangail District. *Studies in family planning*, **17**(1): 13–21 (1986).

22. MOLA, G. & AITKEN, I. Maternal mortality in Papua New Guinea, 1976–1983. *Papua New Guinea medical journal*, **27**(2): 65–71 (1984).

23. FORTNEY, J. Reproductive mortality in two developing countries. *Outlook*, June 1986, pp. 6–7.

24. THOMPSON, B. & BAIRD, D. Some impressions of childbearing in tropical areas. *Journal of obstetrics and gynaecology of the British Commonwealth*, **74**: 329 (1967).

25. MOERMAN, M. L. Growth of the birth canal in adolescent girls. *American journal of obstetrics and gynecology*, **143**(5): 528–532 (1982).

26. PARR, J. H. & RAMSAY, I. The presentation of osteomalacia in pregnancy. *British journal of obstetrics and gynaecology*, **91**: 816–818 (1984).

27. RENDLE-SHORT, C. W. & STEWART, D. B. Pelvic inflammatory

disease. In: Lawson, J. B. & Stewart, D. B., ed. *Obstetrics and gynaecology in the tropics.* London, Edward Arnold, 1967.

28. ADCOCK, L. Uterine rupture experience in Ghana. *Obstetrics and gynaecology*, **22**: 671 (1963).

29. KRISHNA-MENON, M. Rupture of the uterus. *Journal of obstetrics and gynaecology of the British Commonwealth*, **69**: 18–28 (1962).

30. ZUNIGA, G. A. & VASQUEZ, J. A. Ruptura uterina. *Revista médica Hondurena,* **1, 2, 3**: 16 (1962).

31. WHO Technical Report Series, No. 503, 1972 (*Nutritional anaemias*: report of a WHO Group of Experts).

32. ROYSTON, E. The prevalence of nutritional anaemia in women in developing countries: a critical review of available information. *World health statistics quarterly*, **35**: 52–91 (1982).

33. DEMAEYER, E. & ADIELS-TEGMAN, M. The prevalence of anaemia in the world. *World health statistics quarterly*, **38**: 302–316 (1985).

34. HARRISON, K. A. Child bearing, health and social priorities. A survey of 22,774 consecutive births in Zaria, Northern Nigeria. *British journal of obstetrics and gynaecology*, Supplement No. 5 (1985).

35. PRICE, T. G. Preliminary report on maternal deaths in the southern highlands of Tanzania in 1983. *Journal of obstetrics and gynaecology of eastern and central Africa*, **3**: 103–110 (1984).

36. TSEGA, E. Viral hepatitis during pregnancy in Ethiopia. *East African medical journal*, **53**(5): 270–277 (1976).

37. BORHANMANESH, F. ET AL. Viral hepatitis during pregnancy. *Gastroenterology*, **64**: 304–312 (1973).

38. DIAZ SALDANA, J. ET AL. Hepatitis por virus durante el embarazo. *Ginecologia y obstétrica de México*, **43**: 399–404 (1978).

39. KWAST, B. E. & STEVENS, J. A. Viral hepatitis as a major cause of maternal mortality in Addis Ababa, Ethiopia. *International journal of gynaecology and obstetrics*, **25**: 99–106 (1987).

40. CHRISTIE, A. B. ET AL. Pregnancy hepatitis in Libya. *Lancet*, **2**(7990): 827–829 (1976).

41. FARNOT CARDOSO, U. Giving birth is safer now. *World health forum*, **7**(4): 348–354 (1986).

42. WOMEN'S CARE INSTITUTION, BEIJING. The analysis of the maternal mortality in Beijing urban districts from 1959 to 1983. *Beijing medicine*, **8**(2): 80–83 (1985).

43. ZHANG, L. & DING, H. CHINA: Analysis of cause and rate of regional maternal death in 21 provinces, municipalities and autonomous regions. *Chinese journal of obstetrics and gynaecology*, **21**(4): 195–197 (1986).

44. GREENWOOD, A. ET AL. A prospective study of pregnancy in a rural area of the Gambia, West Africa. *Bulletin of the World Health Organization*, **65**(5): 635–644 (1987).

# Chapter 6

# DEATHS FROM ABORTION[1]

Every year between 40 and 60 million women seek termination of an unwanted pregnancy (*1*). Induced abortion is the oldest, and probably still the most widely used method of fertility control. Yet because it touches on some of the most profound religious and moral issues, few societies have been able to look dispassionately at the health aspects of abortion as it affects the woman.

In many parts of the world induced abortion is still illegal or severely restricted by the law; elsewhere some governments that have legalized pregnancy termination have yet to provide adequate services to meet the demand. As a result, a large proportion of the world's women are without access to safe procedures carried out by professionally qualified personnel under aseptic conditions (*2*).

However, there is overwhelming evidence that neither restrictive laws nor lack of access to professional care stop women from seeking abortion. On the contrary, such obstacles affect only the outcome of the procedure. The woman forced to turn secretly to an unqualified back-street abortionist faces a risk of death perhaps 100 to 500 times greater than the woman who has access to a skilled operator and hygienic conditions. This is particularly significant in developing countries where rates of maternal mortality are high.

This chapter will look at the social context of abortion, its legal status and health consequences in different parts of the

---

[1] An abortion is the termination of a pregnancy before the fetus has become capable of independent extra-uterine life. According to medical tradition this covers the first 28 weeks of gestation, counting from the first day of the last normal menstrual period.

An induced abortion is one in which there has been deliberate interference with the pregnancy—either by the woman herself or by someone else—with the aim of terminating it.

All abortions not voluntarily induced are classified as spontaneous, even if an external cause such as trauma, accident or disease is involved. Spontaneous abortion is also known as miscarriage.

world. It will also discuss the costs to the health services of dealing with the complications of illegal induced abortion, and the relationship between abortion and contraception.

## Abortion and the law

Fig. 6.1 shows the legal status of induced abortion in different countries in 1986. While the law sets the scene against which abortion is practised, other factors determine whether or not an individual woman will have a safe professional operation or a hazardous one in the hands of an unskilled abortionist. For the rich and socially advantaged there is always a choice, no matter what the laws of their country, because they can travel abroad if need be. In 1984, for example, 31 300 legal abortions were procured in the United Kingdom by women coming from areas with less liberal abortion laws, mostly in Europe but some as far afield as South Africa and parts of the United States (*3*).

Fig. 6.1. Legal status of abortion throughout the world, according to proportion of the world's population affected

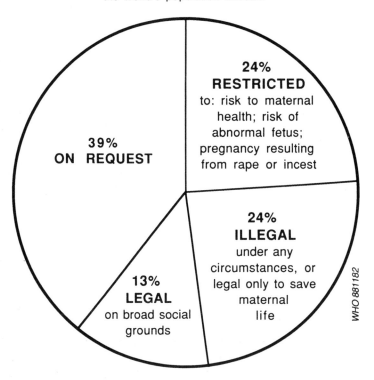

*Source*: Tietze & Henshaw (*3*).

In some countries where laws are restrictive, physicians are nevertheless prepared to perform abortions privately while the authorities turn a blind eye. This is the case, for example, in the Republic of Korea and China (Province of Taiwan). In Cuba abortions were available in public health facilities some years before the operation was legalized in 1979. In Egypt, too, physicians are reported to carry out abortions in large medical centres for reasons that are not permitted by law. It is often the rich and socially advantaged who have access to these safer abortions.

In some countries restrictive laws are loosely interpreted. For example, in Bangladesh, where abortion is only legally permitted to save the life of the pregnant woman, menstrual regulation is part of the national family planning programme and available in health facilities. According to Bangladesh's Institute of Law, menstrual regulation (evacuation of the contents of the uterus by suction) is not covered by the abortion laws because of the fact that pregnancy cannot be established. It states: "Menstrual regulation is now recognised as an interim method of establishing non-pregnancy for the woman who is at risk of being pregnant. Whether or not she is in fact pregnant is no longer an issue" (3).

Conversely, in some countries with few legal restrictions on abortion, many women do not in fact have access to safe procedures. This may be because of a shortage of recognized facilities or qualified operators. The personal antipathy of physicians or administrators towards abortion may also frustrate access, or inhibitions in the women themselves may make them reluctant to go openly to an impersonal government institution for such a purpose. Lack of information, too, leaves many women unaware of the law and their rights under it. A 1971 survey in the Republic of Korea, for instance, found that two-thirds of the respondents had no idea of the legal status of abortion in their country (3).

In India, where abortion has been legal on broad grounds since 1971, registered practitioners are concentrated in urban areas. By 1984 only about 1000 physicians of a total of nearly 15 000 trained to perform abortions were providing the service in rural areas, where 78% of India's people live (3). In 1980 it was established that only 388 000 of the 4–6 million abortions performed in India that year were reported as having been carried out in government health facilities (2, 3). There is considerable under-reporting of abortions carried out in private health facilities, but nevertheless it is evident that illicit abortions are widespread.

In Tunisia, where abortion on demand is legal, one in three is still thought to be carried out illegally by an unqualified operator (3, 4). In Zambia, the only country in sub-Saharan Africa where abortion has been legal on broad social grounds since 1972, evidence from hospital records in 1976 suggests that most women continued to use unqualified practitioners, but that liberalization of the law made them more ready to seek medical treatment if things went wrong. The cumbersome administrative requirements in Zambia possibly act as a deterrent; the law stipulates that a legal abortion must be approved by three physicians including a specialist, and must be performed in hospital unless an emergency makes that impossible (2).

## Death attributed to illegal abortion[1]

Assessing the extent of illegal abortion and its contribution to maternal mortality is almost entirely a matter of guess-work in many countries, since those involved are understandably reluctant to admit to a criminal act, and one that often carries a social stigma. However, even without the full picture it is apparent that criminal abortion constitutes a very serious public health problem (see Table 6.1).

In Latin America, complications of illegal abortion are thought to be the main cause of death in women between the ages of 15 and 39 years (5). Reports from many developing countries cite abortion as one of the main underlying causes of maternal death, if not the main one. For example, a survey of maternal deaths in Addis Ababa between 1981 and 1983 found that 54% of direct obstetric deaths were due to complications following criminal abortion (6). Reports from Colombia,[2] Jamaica (2) and Nigeria (7) have given figures of 29%, 33% and 35% of maternal deaths, respectively.

---

[1] Abortion mortality can be measured in various ways. The abortion mortality rate is the number of deaths attributed to abortion per 100 000 women of reproductive age. The abortion mortality ratio, also known as the death-to-case rate or case-fatality rate, is the number of deaths per 100 000 abortions. However, where abortion is illegal, accurate information about its occurrence is almost impossible to obtain; usually the abortion mortality ratio is based on hospital admissions for abortion complications, and it is generally expressed as the number of deaths per 1000 cases.

[2] Rodriguez, J. et al. Avoidable mortality and maternal mortality in Cali, Colombia. In: *Interregional Meeting on the Prevention of Maternal Mortality, Geneva, 11–15 November 1985.* Unpublished WHO document FHE/PMM/85.9.1.

Table 6.1. Estimated annual number of abortion-related deaths in certain developing regions, about 1980

| Region[a] | Number of women aged 15–44 years (millions) | Assumed rate per million women aged 15–44 | | Estimated number of abortion-related deaths | |
|---|---|---|---|---|---|
| | | Minimum | Maximum | Minimum | Maximum |
| Latin America | 79 | 50 | 50 | 3 950 | 3 950 |
| Africa | 98 | 50 | 500 | 4 900 | 49 000 |
| South-East Asia and Oceania | 81 | 50 | 500 | 4 050 | 40 500 |
| South-West Asia | 20 | 50 | 500 | 1 000 | 10 000 |
| South Asia | 220 | 500 | 500 | 101 000 | 101 000 |
| Total | 480 | — | — | 114 900 | 204 450 |

[a] Data for East Asia are not available.

According to registration data for Romania the proportion was as high as 86% of maternal deaths in 1984.

Looking at abortion mortality from a different perspective, a 1986 report from a rural area of Bangladesh spoke of 2040 women dying per 100 000 illegal operations (8), though this is thought to be an exceptionally high ratio.

The part played by spontaneous abortion in this picture is hard to assess, since it is frequently not differentiated in reports of abortion-related death and rarely studied in its own right.

Most of what is known about abortion-related mortality comes from hospital records, death certificates and community-based surveys (see also Chapter 2). Records from hospitals indicate the number of women admitted for treatment of the complications following criminal abortion and the number of women who subsequently die. Abortion trends can be monitored from fluctuations in the number of admissions. But hospital records are unsatisfactory as baseline data for a number of reasons. They are not always efficiently kept and may therefore be inaccurate. And if the prevailing social and legal climate is against abortion, there will be a tendency to falsify clinical diagnoses and causes of death on the records in order to protect people.

Furthermore, these data represent only the tip of the iceberg since hospitals see only the women with complications who have sought help and been admitted. It is impossible to calculate from this source how many women suffer complications and perhaps die without ever receiving medical care. The picture can be clouded, too, by admission policy. Where hospitals take in only desperately ill women, the death-to-case ratio is far higher than in hospitals that admit women with relatively mild symptoms.

Death certificates are also unsatisfactory as a source of information on abortion-related mortality since many deaths in developing countries are not registered at all. Furthermore, certificates often do not give details of the underlying cause of death, and are particularly unlikely to specify induced abortion where this might lead to involvement with the police and judicial system.

The inadequacy of such data as a basis for assessing countrywide incidence is demonstrated by a systematic evaluation of cause-of-death statistics carried out between 1962 and 1964 by the Pan American Health Organization in ten cities of Latin America (9). Two cities each were studied in Brazil and Colombia and one each in Argentina, Chile, Guatemala, Mexico, Peru and Venezuela. Because burial regulations were strictly enforced in these cities, reporting of deaths was assumed to be virtually complete. In each city the investigators selected a sample of death certificates of people aged between 15 and 44 years and sought additional information from hospitals, attending physicians, and the families of the deceased.

According to the original death certificates, 132 deaths in the sample drawn from the ten cities were attributed to abortion complications. The review procedure increased this total by a half, to 198 deaths overall. For individual cities the increases resulting from the review ranged from 11% for Santiago to 229% for Bogotá (see Table 6.2).

Table 6.2. Maternal mortality in 10 Latin American cities, 1962–64

| City | Proportion of maternal mortality that was due to abortion (%) |
|---|---|
| Bogotá | 37 |
| Cali | 37 |
| Caracas | 46 |
| Guatemala City | 47 |
| La Plata | 23 |
| Lima | 13 |
| Mexico City | 20 |
| Santiago | 53 |
| São Paulo | 20 |
| Ribeiro Preto | 19 |

Source: Puffer & Wynne Griffith (9).

Community-based surveys have the advantage of shedding light on what goes on outside hospital walls. They allow for a more realistic assessment of the incidence of illegal abortion and the frequency of complications. However, eliciting accurate and complete information about so personal and sensitive a matter is extremely difficult. Surveys in China (Province of Taiwan), the Philippines, the Republic of Korea, and Thailand, found that rates of abortion revealed by questioning abortion providers were consistently higher than those revealed by questioning women themselves about their reproductive behaviour (2). It is often difficult to identify the abortion providers for questioning.

## Factors affecting the risk of death from abortion

The risk associated with induced abortion depends on:

— the method used;

— the competence of the abortionist;

— the stage of pregnancy at which the operation is performed;

— the age and general health of the pregnant woman;

— the availability and quality of medical care if anything should go wrong.

While legal medical abortion is now one of the safest surgical procedures, the risk of suffering serious complications and perhaps death is considerable where the operation is performed by an unqualified abortionist under unhygienic conditions.

The stage of pregnancy at which a woman seeks abortion is one of the most important factors affecting risk. A study of 1890 women in Santiago, Chile, for example, found that 47% of those who had undergone abortion in the third to fifth month of pregnancy ended up in hospital compared with 18% of those who had been aborted during the first month (10). And in the United States it has been calculated that the risk of death associated with legal abortions carried out in the first eight weeks of pregnancy is more than 20 times lower than the risk involved in giving birth (2). Even with legal abortion, however, the risk of death rises with each additional week of gestation (see Table 6.3).

Unfortunately, for various reasons many women overstep the safest period for termination, even where abortion is legal. Lack of information or access to the "system", as well as legal and procedural delays, are common obstacles to timely abortion, as is difficulty in finding money to pay an abortionist, whether legal or illegal. In the case of very young unmarried girls in the majority of cultures, shame and the

Table 6.3. Number of deaths per 100 000 legal abortions, by week of gestation, USA, 1977–81

| Weeks of gestation | Deaths per 100 000 legal abortions |
|---|---|
| 8 or less | 0.4 |
| 9–10 | 0.6 |
| 11–12 | 0.8 |
| 13–15 | 1.2 |
| 16–20 | 7.1 |

*Source:* Tietze & Henshaw (*3*)

fear of social isolation often inhibit them from seeking an early solution to an unwanted pregnancy.

As already noted, all the evidence points to the fact that making abortion illegal does not stop the practice; it only makes it more dangerous. The extra risk associated with its illegal status will vary from country to country, but the experience of some countries that have changed their laws illustrates the impact that liberalization can have, especially if it goes hand in hand with a commitment to make legal abortion services widely available.

This was the case in Singapore where the abortion laws were liberalized in 1970 in response to the high mortality associated with illegal operations. In 1974 the law was liberalized further, making abortion available on demand up to 24 weeks (*11*). The number of known abortion cases for the period 1968–70 was 11 151, of which 51 died, whereas 26 died out of 40 880 known abortion cases for the period 1974–76 (*2, 11*). The marked decline in deaths was attributed to fewer illegal abortions.

By contrast, Romania experienced a sharp increase in abortion-related deaths after it tightened a previously liberal law in November 1966 (see Fig. 6.2). The figure rose from 64 deaths in 1965 to 432 in 1976, and 449 in 1984. By 1972–73 hospital admissions in Bucharest for complications following illegal abortion were running at about one-third of the number of legal abortions performed before 1966 (*12*).

In Cuba, where abortion on demand is now legal and has been widely available in hospitals for a long time, the mortality ratio for hospital abortions averaged 1.0 per 100 000

Fig. 6.2.   Effects of the introduction in Romania, in November 1966, of an anti-abortion law

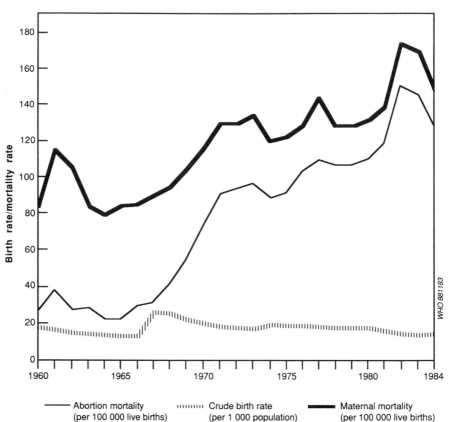

procedures for the period 1968–74 (*2*). In the United States in 1981 only 7 deaths were attributed to legal abortion out of a total of 1 577 300 procedures (*3*).

## Incidence of abortion[1]

It is estimated that, each year, worldwide, 40–70 per 1000 women of reproductive age have an abortion, and that

---

[1] The following different measurements are used in relation to abortion. The abortion rate is the number of abortions relative to a specified population over a period of time, usually one year. It is often expressed as a number of abortions per 1000 women of reproductive age. The abortion ratio, on the other hand, is the number of abortions relative to specified events such as live births or pregnancies over a given period of time. This, too, is often expressed as a number of abortions per 1000 events. The prevalence, generally expressed as a percentage, refers to the proportion of women who have had an abortion during their lifetime.

between one-fifth and one-third of all pregnancies are terminated[1] (see Fig. 6.3).

It appears that, in the short term, liberalizing a previously restrictive law increases the total number of induced abortions. This is largely because it offers a choice to women who would otherwise give birth rather than risk a backstreet operation, coupled with the fact that, with its criminal status removed, abortion is used more readily in the case of contraceptive failure. However, the effect is two-pronged. At the same time that there is an increase in abortions, there is also a marked decline in the number of deaths because of the greater safety of legal abortions.

Economic development also appears to have a complex effect on abortion. If it is associated with a decline in breast-feeding (which is a natural inhibitor of fertility) then it tends to increase the proportion of women able to conceive. Development tends to provide better education and employment prospects for women, thereby increasing the motivation to postpone or limit childbearing. The better health care and living conditions that may come in the wake of development also tend to decrease pressure for a couple to have many children, since more of them are likely to survive to adulthood.

Furthermore, development is commonly associated with the drift of rural people to the cities in search of a better standard of living, and this also tends to increase pressure for family planning, in that children who may be an economic necessity in the countryside can become a burden in an overcrowded urban slum, at least until they are old enough to go out to work themselves. Moreover, the disintegration of traditional rural communities as people move into the cities commonly leads to a relaxation of social controls over sexual behaviour, and to higher rates of unwanted pregnancy. All these changes associated with development— unless they are accompanied by better knowledge of, and access to, family planning methods—tend to increase the incidence of induced abortion, and thereby the number of abortion-related deaths.

On the other hand, economic and social development tends to improve nutrition and health standards, thus increasing women's resistance to infection and other complications of

[1] *Health and status of women.* Unpublished WHO document FHE/80.1.

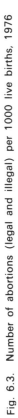

Fig. 6.3. Number of abortions (legal and illegal) per 1000 live births, 1976

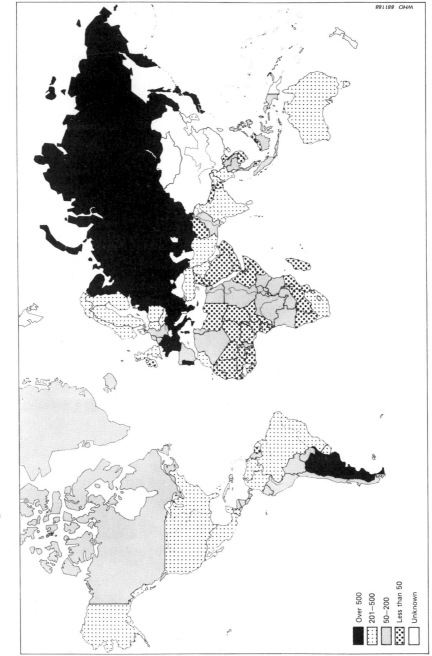

WHO 881188

Over 500
201–500
50–200
Less than 50
Unknown

*Source: People, 3: 18 (1978).*

abortion. Development also tends to improve the availability and quality of medical services which, as well as reducing the incidence of serious complications, improves the chances of survival if such complications do occur.

## Regional trends

In this most obscure field of public health, data from various sources nevertheless give some idea of the trends in different parts of the world.

### Latin America

Based on the results of a survey of data from 19 countries, it has been estimated that around 3.4 million abortions are performed each year in Latin America, i.e., 45 per 1000 women of reproductive age (5), though the International Planned Parenthood Federation had earlier suggested that the rate was around 65 per 1000 (2). Speaking of Santiago, Chile, one observer noted: "Between 10% and 30% of beds in obstetric and gynaecological wards of most Latin American hospitals are filled by women suffering abortion complications." Furthermore, the same observer said that on the evidence of research: "The Catholic church undoubtedly still plays an important role in helping to maintain restrictive abortion legislation and in attempting to ensure that abortion services are unavailable, yet the church appears to have little or no practical influence on the attitudes of individual women with unwanted pregnancy" (13).

### Sub-Saharan Africa

Very little information on abortion has come out of Africa, with the result that there are no reliable estimates of how widely it is practised. Hospital admissions for abortion complications will be the very tip of the iceberg in many African countries since a very large proportion of people still live beyond the reach of modern health services. However, reports from Zimbabwe estimate that around 28% of maternal deaths are abortion-related (31), while estimates for the United Republic of Tanzania (32) and Addis Ababa (6) put the figures at around 21% and 54% respectively. Because of the huge gaps in information, such figures indicate little more than that illegal abortion is a major killer of women in their childbearing years. Zambia is the only African country in which abortion is legal.

## Asia

The incidence of induced abortion is generally considered to be high in most Asian countries, regardless of its legal status. For example, the rate in 1978 for Seoul, Republic of Korea, where it is legally restricted, was estimated from a survey of providers to be 235 per 1000 married women aged between 15 and 44 years (*3*). The rate for Thailand, where the abortion laws are also restrictive, was calculated in 1978 at 37 per 1000 women of reproductive age, with a ratio of 245 abortions per 1000 live births, while Singapore, where abortion is legal, reported a rate of 28.4 per 1000 women of reproductive age in 1981, and a ratio of 371 per 1000 live births in 1976. In India, where it is legal but government services are unevenly spread, the IPPF estimated a rate of 55 illegal abortions per 1000 women aged 15 to 44 years for 1970, while the comparable rate for legal abortions in 1983 was only 3.3 per 1000 (*3*).

## North Africa and the Eastern Mediterranean countries

Abortion laws in this area tend to be highly restrictive in line with Muslim tradition and the high value placed on female chastity. Tunisia is an exception. Abortion on request has been available there for women with five children or more since 1965, and for all women during the first trimester since 1973 (*3*). Turkey has recently followed suit.

Strict rules and taboos surrounding sexual matters mean that little reliable recent information is available on abortion incidence in most of the countries in this area. However, records show that in many urban hospitals in Egypt there are half as many admissions for abortion complications as for deliveries, and in parts of Iraq abortion admissions may even exceed deliveries (*12*). A survey of women in Lebanon in 1961 found, on the women's own evidence, that, in country villages, around 0.2% of pregnancies were terminated, whereas the figure was 8–14% in urban areas (*12*). In Tunisia the rate of abortion for 1974, the first year it was legal, rose to 10.9 per 1000 women aged 15 to 44. In 1982 it reached 17.2 and then dropped to 13.6 in 1985 (*3*).

## Characteristics of women seeking abortion

There is a wide variety of reasons and personal circumstances under which women seek abortion. Everywhere the pattern shifts constantly with changes in the prevailing social, legal and moral climate. However, some broad general characteristics of abortion-seekers can be identified.

In many places less is known about illegal abortion at the wealthier levels of society than at any other level, since those with money are far more likely to be able to procure an abortion from a skilled operator in a sanitary environment. They will be less likely to suffer complications or die as a result and the fact of their abortion will therefore not appear in hospital records or civil registration data.

As a general rule induced abortion is more common among city dwellers than among rural people. A survey in Malaysia, for instance, found abortion to be four times more frequent in urban than in rural women. And in Alexandria, Egypt, it is estimated to be three times as frequent (*14*). Reports from Latin America and Africa also confirm this tendency. (However, in some places the picture may be distorted by the fact that women in urban areas can get to hospital more easily in the event of complications, whereas the fate of those beyond the reach of the health system generally remains unknown.) Apart from the greater motivation for abortion in the urban setting discussed earlier, this difference may reflect a greater concentration of services, legal and illegal, in the cities, and more freedom to take such a step in the relative anonymity of the city.

Several trends have been observed in abortion among unmarried women—a phenomenon that appears to be increasingly common wherever traditional moral codes are giving way to greater sexual freedom, particularly with the drift to the cities. For instance, studies carried out as long ago as 1968–71 in some capital cities of Latin America — Asunción, Bogotá, Lima, Panama City, and Buenos Aires— found that though teenagers had the lowest rate of abortion, the rate was rising more rapidly than in any other age group (*15*). Furthermore, a survey by the International Fertility Research Programme (IFRP) of hospital admissions for abortion complications in nine Latin American countries between 1974 and 1979 revealed that 18% of cases were unmarried women (*2*).

Though abortion among married women with children is the more common pattern in Asian countries, reports of surveys from the Republic of Korea and Thailand suggest that the incidence among unmarried women in those countries is now quite high. The latter tend to be students or working women anxious to avoid disrupting their studies or employment. Certain other groups of women particularly vulnerable to unwanted pregnancy are also likely to seek termination. A study in Thailand, for instance, found that 92% of a sample of 180 girls who worked in massage parlours had had induced abortions (*12*).

Many reports indicate a strong positive correlation with education, induced abortion being considerably more common among unmarried women with secondary education, or higher, than among those with no education. This trend is evident in sub-Saharan Africa, where abortion is, at present, more common among young unmarried urban women than among any other group, and is thought to indicate a desire to postpone marriage and childbearing in the interests of education and employment. According to many reports, a high proportion of those seeking abortion are still in school. A survey in Nigeria, for instance, found that only 12 of the 45 schools surveyed had been unaffected by pregnancy among students. The pregnant students had been expelled from school or withdrawn by their families, or they had died as a result of abortion (*16*).

An important aspect of this sad picture is that teenagers rarely have access to contraception, even where there is every likelihood of early sexual experience. In Ghana and the United Republic of Tanzania, for instance, family planning is directed at married people only. Besides, very young women are the least likely to have information about abortion or the financial means to procure a relatively safe, if illegal, operation. They are therefore most vulnerable to complications and death.

Induced abortion may also be used by married women anxious to postpone childbearing. In a field study carried out in Malaysia between 1973 and 1974, about one-third of the respondents gave this explanation for seeking abortion (*2*). An IFRP hospital-based study in Latin America in 1980 revealed that, unlike the pattern in earlier years, the majority of married women treated for complications of induced abortion were in their 20s, and about 25% of them had no living children (*17*). This was the case, too, in a 1973 hospital-based study in Thailand, which found that a high proportion of the married women who had induced abortions were childless. In Chile there is evidence of a high rate of abortion among domestic servants, who tend to live in the houses of their employers where servants' children are not welcome (15).

In some regions the women who seek abortion are predominantly married, with several children already, and are using abortion to terminate childbearing rather than as a means of postponing or spacing births. Frequently such women are from poor families with a limited tradition of family planning and contraception. For instance, in Greece, where contraception was illegal until 1980, induced abortion (also illegal but easier to obtain than contraceptives) became widespread as a means of limiting families, especially in cities where housing was in short supply (18).

In Latin America, studies have shown that the rate of abortion among women over 35 is twice that for women aged 20–34, and that the rate among women with five or more children is over 2.5 times that among women with only one child (13). In Tunisia in 1976 three out of every five women who sought legal termination had previously given birth four times or more (4).

An analysis of 500 women seeking legal abortion at a family planning centre in Allahabad, India, revealed that the vast majority were married, aged 20–29 and most had several children already. Among the urban women in the survey 45% had one or two children and 32% had three or four children, while among rural women 20% had one or two children, 26% had three or four children, and 41% more than five children (19).

In some regions abortion appears to be socially acceptable and used frequently as a method of fertility control. This is the case in China. In the USSR, where the stated aim of the law is to give women "the possibility to decide for themselves the question of motherhood", there are estimated to be about twice as many induced abortions as live births (3) (though figures vary considerably between regions and ethnic groups). One report in 1970 in the USSR revealed that of 1350 women interviewed, 70% had had two or more abortions, and 12% had had more than six (12). A study of induced abortion in Yugoslavia found that many women were choosing abortion rather than contraception for a number of complex psychological reasons, including the need constantly to prove fertility, because a woman's self-image, social status and power are closely related to procreation (20). It was suggested that this pattern was largely a function of inequality between men and women, so it is likely that this attitude to abortion would be found in some other societies with similar social structures.

## Methods of induced abortion

Methods used to induce abortion in developing countries run the gamut from advanced medical techniques used by physicians, to the age-old and often harmful techniques used by traditional healers, helpful neighbours or the pregnant women themselves.

Of the methods used by physicians and health workers (usually within a legal framework), "instrumental evacuation", primarily by means of dilatation and curettage (D & C) is the most common. D & C involves dilating the cervical canal to allow the insertion of surgical instruments for removing the contents of the uterus. Surgical curettage is being progressively replaced by suction curettage, of which menstrual regulation[1] is a variant.

Although instrumental evacuation, including menstrual regulation, is mainly used by physicians, reports from all regions indicate that it is also used by other health workers at all levels of the health care system. Carried out by skilled personnel in the first trimester of pregnancy, this is considered to be the safest method of abortion.

Hysterotomy, a major surgical operation requiring admission to hospital for several days, is in essence a caesarean section before the fetus is viable. Hysterotomy has been virtually abandoned in developed countries because it carries a high risk of complications and death. Yet in spite of its dubious record elsewhere, it is an accepted procedure for legal terminations in India, where it is almost invariably combined with surgical sterilization (3).

Another procedure, which is used during the second trimester of pregnancy and generally within a legal hospital setting, is the stimulation of uterine contractions by the introduction of

---

[1] Menstrual regulation, also referred to as endometrial aspiration, minisuction, interception of pregnancy, or occasionally atraumatic uterine evacuation, is a procedure in which a small tube (cannula) is inserted into the uterus and the uterine contents removed by a vacuum syringe connected to the outer end, or by a small pump operated either manually or by an electric motor. The procedure should be limited to the first two weeks after a missed menstrual period, when pregnancy cannot yet be reliably diagnosed.

a saline solution or prostaglandin to the uterus. From beginning to end the procedure generally takes 36–72 hours to complete. Severe vomiting and diarrhoea are frequent side-effects from the irritant action of the prostaglandins, and the procedure is not always effective the first time.

Introduction of fluids into the uterus in the hope of inducing abortion is common practice among unqualified abortionists and among women trying to abort themselves. The fluid may be anything from soapy water to household disinfectant introduced via a syringe or douche bag.

In some countries abortifacient pastes containing irritants intended for use in the same way have been reported as being advertised in medical journals aimed at the general practitioner (i.e., for the purpose of clandestine, illegal abortion). In India these pastes have been banned by the government, but are still being sold over the counter.

Oral preparations are also common, and a wide range of herbs and medicines believed to be abortifacients can be found on market stalls in developing countries. Indeed there is a flourishing worldwide trade in such products, trading on the back of desperation and superstition (21).

In Bangladesh such a preparation might contain quinine, potassium permanganate, ergot or mercury (22), while in Malaysia pills made from lead oxide and olive oil are sold (12). In India dried carrot tops for infusion are seen on market stalls, and in the Philippines an infusion of banana and local *kalachulchi* leaves is sold for the same purpose (12).

One book (12) gives a vivid picture of this trade in a description of "one of the most curious sites for the sale of abortifacients"—the Quiapo in central Manila: "The Quiapo is the busiest and most loved church in Manila. Mass is celebrated in relays from 6.30 a.m. on Sundays and the church is crowded for many hours, with hundreds standing in the aisles. Immediately outside the church—in physical contact with its walls—are rows of booths. They sell three things: religious pictures, candles and herbal remedies (of which those for late periods are the most important). A bottle of abortifacient medicine (always sold in the local San Miguel beer bottle) costs 1.50 pesos (25 US cents). An average stall sells about 20 bottles on a Sunday to women going to, or leaving, mass. There are 40–50 stalls clinging to the walls of the Quiapo. The whole is a vivid demonstration that neither the congregation nor priests perceive the intent to terminate a very early pregnancy as a sin".

Another method of inducing abortion used widely by illegal abortionists or pregnant women themselves is the introduction of foreign bodies into the uterus. In Ghana, two types of twig are commonly used (*12*). One, the dried stem of the *commelina* plant, when inserted into the uterus, takes up moisture and swells, dilating the cervix and causing abortion. The other, which comes from the *jatropha* plant, contains a corrosive chemical which combines with the effect of the jatropha twig, as a foreign body, to cause abortion.

In parts of Latin America illegal abortionists sometimes insert one end of a flexible catheter into the uterus, taping the other end to the inside of the woman's thigh, and instructing her to walk about so that the catheter disturbs the contents of the womb. A study in Santiago, Chile, found this to be the most hazardous method of all (*10*). But the words of a doctor on the septic ward of the Materno-Infantil maternity hospital in Bogotá, Colombia, show that desperate women face all manner of dangers from back-street abortions (*23*): "A few of the *señoras* use traditional methods such as quinine water—preparations that are either poisonous to the woman as well as the fetus, or useless. The majority use a hollow rubber or plastic tube and poke through it with things like umbrella spokes, knitting needles, or even sticks and bits of wire. As a result, we get women in here with ruptured wombs, rectums, intestines, bladders. One girl came in with her womb, intestines and kidneys slashed as if she had been carved up with a kitchen knife. The conditions of cleanliness are subhuman. There is no disinfectant or sterilisation. Septicaemia, abscesses, peritonitis are common consequences, and most of our patients have to have their womb or ovaries removed. This is often a terrible tragedy for them because from then on they think of themselves as incomplete, and their husbands may no longer consider them a whole woman. Many couples have broken up because of this".

In some countries, particularly in South-East Asia, Africa and the Eastern Mediterranean countries, non-invasive methods such as abortion by massage are very commonly used, and are often accompanied by infusions. This involves pressure on the stomach of the pregnant woman by the abortionist using her hands, or even her feet, long enough to induce bleeding. The procedure can cause damage to the internal organs and internal bleeding.

## The main complications and causes of death

As already mentioned, the risks of complications or death following legal abortion are extremely slight compared with those of illegal, unskilled abortion. Differing mortality and morbidity rates between countries largely reflect differences in the general health status of the women involved and the average stage of pregnancy at which abortion is performed, which is the most important single factor. The following discussion therefore applies mainly to complications following illegal, unskilled abortion.

The most frequent early complication under these conditions is sepsis caused by incomplete abortion, i.e., part or all of the products of conception are retained in the uterus. If the infection is not treated, it can become generalized to produce what is known as septic abortion, which is the most common fatal complication of illegal abortion. Septic abortion can also be the result of incomplete spontaneous abortion, though this is rare.

The most serious infections, rarely seen in developed countries today, are those involving anaerobic bacteria found in soil and manure, which cause gas gangrene or tetanus. They are almost invariably the result of using dirty instruments.

If septic abortion is caused by a particularly virulent organism and is left untreated, the patient may develop septic shock, an extremely grave condition in which the circulation slows down and organs of the body are thereby starved of oxygen. Before abortion was legalized in the United States, the proportion of septic abortions that led to septic shock was between 1.8% and 3.8%; in Egypt in 1973 the corresponding proportion was 15.6% of a sample of 141 septic abortion cases seen in hospital (2). Records from a hospital in Madurai, India, showed that 10.25% of patients with septic abortion developed septic shock (2).

After sepsis, the next most frequently reported cause of death following illegal abortion is haemorrhage. Haemorrhage may be due to incomplete abortion, or to injury of the pelvic organs or intestines, and death is frequently the result of lack of blood or equipment for transfusion in the hospital.

127

Other potentially fatal complications of induced abortion are
blockages in the circulatory system caused by blood clots, air
bubbles or fluid; severe disturbances of the blood-clotting
mechanism (disseminated intravascular coagulation) caused by
overwhelming infections; and poisoning from abortifacient
medicines resulting in kidney failure.

For those who survive the early complications of unskilled
abortion there may be long-term adverse effects. For
example, infections can lead to blockages in, or permanent
damage to, the fallopian tubes, with consequent infertility.
Tubal problems are the leading cause of infertility in many
developing countries, occurring in 73% of a sample of
infertile women in Nairobi, Kenya, and 62% and 56%,
respectively, of comparable samples in Indonesia and Tunisia
(24). It is not possible to determine what proportion of such
cases result from abortion, or what proportion might have
been caused by pelvic inflammatory disease associated with
sexually transmitted diseases or unhygienic obstetric practice.
However, in Greece, abortion is believed to be the main
cause of tubal infertility (18). Ectopic pregnancy is another
possible consequence of infection involving the fallopian
tubes.

Infertility is a tragic consequence of abortion for the young
woman who has not yet started a family, particularly in
cultures where the ability to have children is highly valued
and the childless woman is pitied or even ostracized.

## Costs to the health services

The complications of abortion are an enormous drain on the
health services. Repairing the damage of illegal abortion
often requires surgery, blood transfusion, antibiotics and a
long stay in hospital for the sick woman.

A survey in Santiago, Chile, found that 40% of all emergency admissions to hospital were for abortion, and it is
estimated that throughout Latin America 10–30% of the
obstetric and gynaecological beds in hospitals are currently
filled with women suffering from the effects of abortion (13).

The picture is similar in other parts of the world. In the
Mama Yemo hospital in Kinshasa, for example, around 60%
of all gynaecological cases were reported to be abortion
complications, while in one hospital in Accra the comparable
rate was over 50% (12). At the same hospital 60–80% of all

minor surgery was for abortion complications, which also accounted for half the hospital's supply of blood for transfusion.

One hospital in Port of Spain, Trinidad, was so overwhelmed by emergency admissions, which included a significant proportion of abortion cases, that it was unable to perform any routine gynaecological operations for eight months during 1971 (*12*).

A study in a hospital in Turkey in the mid-1970s found that the cost of treating complications following an unskilled operation was about four times the cost of performing a medical abortion (*2*). Blood transfusion was the single most expensive item of treatment, accounting for 49% of the total cost. This seems to be the general rule, and since blood is often in short supply in hospitals in the developing world, illegal abortion puts a double burden on resources.

The cost of occupying hospital beds can be considerable too. A Santiago hospital reported that during six months of 1974 the cost of beds for illegal abortion cases was US$ 23 690. It was later estimated that if these illegal abortions had been legal medical terminations, the saving in bed occupancy alone would have been around US$ 20 576 (*2*).

In the early 1970s a pilot project conducted in Chile furnished impressive evidence of the relative costs of legal and illegal abortion to the health services (*12*). For a brief period abortion was approved as a medical procedure in a selected area of Santiago, and Chilean physicians performed a total of 3250 abortions during the period of the study. There was no publicity but, as word spread, the demand for the hospital service increased until a ratio of one abortion for every two births was reached. At the same time admissions for complications of illegal abortion showed a marked decline. Careful analysis of the results showed that the saving achieved by replacing a high proportion of dangerous back-street abortions with medical terminations was approximately US$ 200 000.

## Abortion and contraception

Because abortion and contraception are both methods by which women avoid unwanted births, it is frequently assumed that the way to eliminate altogether the evils of illegal

abortion is to make contraceptives widely available. Unfortunately, the moral and political dilemmas associated with
legalizing abortion are not so simply avoided. Encouraging
the informed and effective use of contraceptives undoubtedly
has the potential to reduce the number of women seeking
abortion, especially among those with a poor history of
contraceptive practice. But it will never eliminate unwanted
pregnancy completely.

One expert has illustrated this point by looking at two
different paths to the same goal: the reduction of fertility
from an average of seven births per woman to an average of
two. He estimated that to achieve this goal in the absence of
contraceptives each woman would require an average of nine
or ten abortions in her lifetime. If, on the other hand,
couples were to use a 95%-effective contraceptive method,
seven out of ten women would require one abortion at some
point in their lives (*25*).

The relationship between contraception and abortion is
extremely complex and a variety of different patterns has
been observed. A simple correlation between increased use
of contraceptives and a decrease in the number of women
admitted to hospital for complications of abortion was
observed in a study in Santiago, Chile (*13*). In 1964 a family
planning programme started in a working-class district of·
town offering free insertion of an IUD to any woman who
had at least one child. The number of acceptances increased
from 4073 in 1964 to 10 271 in 1968, with a total over the
five years of 36 418. Over the same period, hospitalization for
abortion complications declined by 29.4% in the study area,
while the trend in Chile as a whole was upwards.

This pattern appears to have held true on a wider scale, too.
As contraceptives became increasingly available throughout
Chile over the next decade, their use is estimated to have
increased rapidly, and to have curbed the practice of
abortion to a significant degree (*2*) (see Fig. 6.4).

Another pattern that has been observed is a positive
relationship between contraception and abortion; under some
circumstances, an active family planning programme goes
hand in hand with higher rates of illegal abortion. This
positive relationship is, in general, most marked at the point
when society first begins to accept the need to limit reproduction; that is, during the demographic transition. This is at
least partly due to the fact that individuals often feel pres-

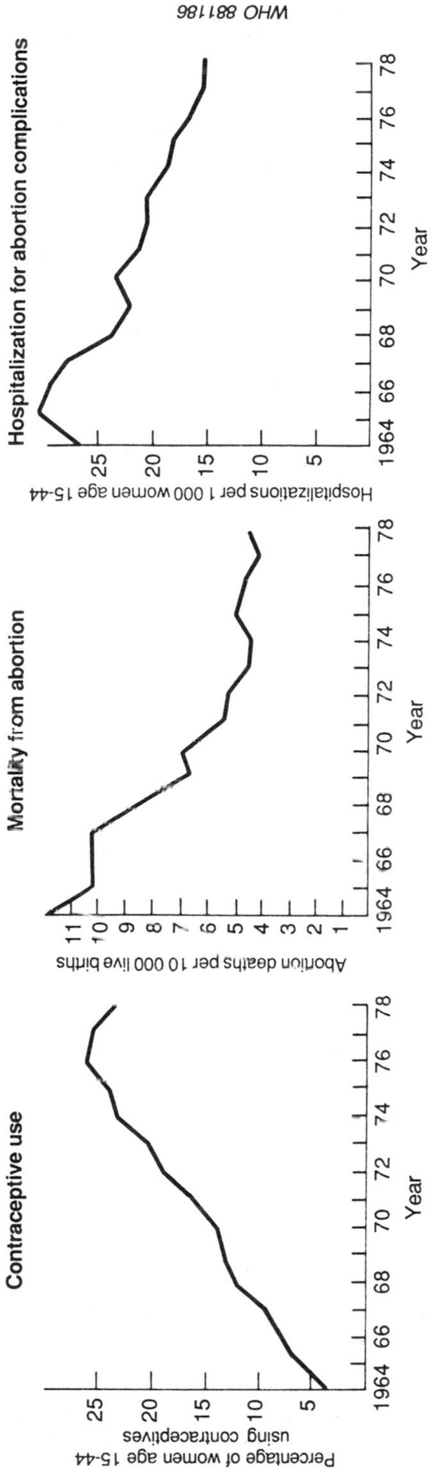

Fig. 6.4. Rates of contraceptive use, abortion mortality and hospitalizations for abortion complications, Chile, 1964–1978

**Contraceptive use**

Percentage of women age 15-44 using contraceptives

**Mortality from abortion**

Abortion deaths per 10 000 live births

**Hospitalization for abortion complications**

Hospitalizations per 1 000 women age 15-44

WHO 881186

sure to limit their family size before effective and acceptable contraceptives are available to them, or they have learnt to use them effectively. Secondly, abortion is used as a back-up in case of contraceptive failure. No method of contraception other than sterilization is absolutely reliable even when used responsibly. Besides, many methods require forethought and a good deal of motivation, so failures of contraception are inevitable. Not surprisingly, perhaps, reports from many countries show that women who have some experience of contraceptive use are more likely to have abortions—whether legal or illegal—than women who have none (26).

The experiences of the Republic of Korea and China (Province of Taiwan) illustrate well the positive relationship between abortion and contraception (12). Both introduced national family planning programmes when the birth rate was still high, and over subsequent years the increasing desire to limit their families made women turn to one or other "method" to achieve this goal.

The family planning programme in the Republic of Korea started in 1962 and in 1966 30% of the country's health budget was devoted to it. During the early years of intense promotion of contraception, the number of women aged 20–44 who admitted that they had undergone induced abortion increased significantly, approximately doubling between 1964 and 1968 (27). The decline in the birth rate between 1960 and 1968 was approximately 30%, of which a significant proportion can be attributed to abortion, since the number of pregnancies reported to have ended in abortion increased from around 5.6% of the total in 1960 to 21.3% in 1968 (12).

In China (Province of Taiwan), the proportion of married women between the ages of 22 and 39 years who had ever used contraceptives increased from 28%′ in 1965, at the beginning of the family planning drive, to 76% in 1976, while the proportion of women who admitted having undergone abortion also rose, from 9% to 21% during the same period (28).

Evidence from several countries, including those of the developed world, indicates that this pattern changes with time. Many countries experienced a similar pattern of rising abortion rates concurrent with increasing use of contraceptives during the early years of family planning programmes, but found that as contraceptives became more readily available and better understood by people, the abortion rates began to fall (*12*).

It seems that this sequence of events is extremely difficult to alter. One opinion is that avoiding a rise in the abortion rate during the demographic transition would require a greater commitment of resources than any national family planning programme has yet contemplated (*12*).

In some countries, people have felt the pressure to control their fertility in the absence of strong family planning services and easily available contraceptives. Under such circumstances the abortion rate is high. This is the picture in Greece, where contraceptives were illegal until 1980 and are still not widely available (*29*), and in Romania, where the birth rate is low and contraceptives are not widely used (*26*). In Romania this appears to be the result of a traditional reliance on abortion to control fertility (despite changes in the abortion laws) and an official restriction on some forms of contraception since 1966.

It is sometimes argued that liberalizing abortion laws will lead to less widespread or irresponsible use of contraception, but there does not appear to be any evidence to support this view. Besides, such a hypothesis would seem to underestimate the personal suffering generally caused by unwanted pregnancy and its consequences. In fact, abortion seems to increase the demand for contraceptives, and research in many countries shows that women are most receptive to contraceptive counselling immediately following abortion.

One study of 2230 women hospitalized for abortion or its complications in India, for example, showed that while only 25% had used any form of contraception before, 88% started to use contraceptives after their abortion (*2*). A comparable study in Thailand of 301 women who had had abortions found that 4% had used contraception before, and 44% subsequently became users (*2*).

Unfortunately, in many areas the health services fail to take advantage of the situation, and women leave hospital after an abortion either without having received family planning counselling or without the possibility of obtaining the contraceptives they want. Where abortion remains illegal, women are doubly disadvantaged; they are unlikely to get guidance on contraception from an illegal abortionist, and therefore remain vulnerable to repeated unwanted pregnancies and dangerous, illegal abortions.

Widespread access to information about contraception and supplies of contraceptives is vitally important in the battle to prevent the tragic loss of life associated with illegal induced abortion. However, as noted above, contraception cannot altogether eliminate the need for abortion. They are two faces of the same coin and, as one observer comments: "If mortality is the sole criterion for judging [a family planning programme's] merits, we may conclude that perfectly safe but not entirely effective contraception—such as the diaphragm or condom—combined with legally induced abortions entails the lowest risk" (*26*).

## Conclusion

Any serious attempt to bring down the rate of maternal mortality cannot avoid confronting the issue of abortion. It is not an unpredictable, aberrant event, but an integral part of the picture of fertility control, and the oldest method in the world. Abortion occurs in liberal and illiberal societies, and the aspect of the operation that is most affected by the society's attitude and the law is the degree of risk it involves.

In the modern world most of the women faced with an unwanted pregnancy will also face a society unwilling to acknowledge their plight or to offer them a safe solution. As a result, many millions find their own solution in the back streets, often at enormous risk to themselves. Procuring an illegal abortion is frequently a lonely, desperate decision and many pay with their lives.

## References

1. HENSHAW, S. K. Induced abortion: a worldwide perspective. *Family planning perspectives*, **18**(6) 250–254 (1986).
2. LISKIN, L. S. Complications of abortion in developing countries. *Population reports*, Series F, No. 7 (1980).
3. TIETZE, C. & HENSHAW, S. K. *Induced abortion. A world review.* 6th ed. New York, Alan Guttmacher Institute, 1986.
4. POPULATION CRISIS COMMITTEE. World abortion trends. *Population*, No. 9 (1982).
5. VIEL, B. Illegal abortion in Latin America. *IPPF medical bulletin*, **16**(4): 1–2 (1982).

6. KWAST, B. E. ET AL. Maternal mortality in Addis Ababa, Ethiopia. *Studies in family planning*, **17**(6): 288–301 (1986).

7. OMU, A. L. ET AL. Adolescent induced abortion in Benin City, Nigeria. *International journal of gynaecology and obstetrics*, **19**(6): 495–499 (1981).

8. KHAN, A. R. ET AL. Induced abortion in a rural area of Bangladesh. *Studies in family planning*, **17**(2): 95–99 (1986).

9. PUFFER, R. R. & WYNNE GRIFFITH, G. *Patterns of urban mortality.* Washington, Pan American Health Organization, 1967 (PAHO Scientific Publication No. 151).

10. ARMIJO, R. & MONREAL, T. Factors associated with complications following provoked abortions. *Journal of sex research*, **4**(1): 1–6 (1968).

11. LIM, L. S. ET AL. Abortion deaths in Singapore (1968–1976). *Singapore medical journal*, **20**(3): 391–394 (1979).

12. POTTS, M. ET AL. *Abortion.* Cambridge, Cambridge University Press, 1977.

13. VIEL, B. The health consequences of illegal abortion in Latin America. In: Zatuchni, G. et al. *Pregnancy termination: procedures, safety and new developments.* London, Harper and Row, 1979.

14. TOPPOZADA, H. K. Epidemiology of abortion in Alexandria. *Alexandria medical journal*, **26**(1,2): 1–167 (1980).

15. PAN AMERICAN HEALTH ORGANIZATION. *Epidemiology of abortion and practices of fertility regulation in Latin America: selected reports.* Washington, 1975 (PAHO Scientific Publication, No. 306).

16. AKINGBA, J. B. Abortion, maternity and other health problems in Nigeria. *Nigerian medical journal*, 7(4): 465–471 (1977).

17. INTERNATIONAL FERTILITY RESEARCH PROGRAM. *Abortion in Latin America.* Triangle Park, NC, 1980 (IFRP Research Report DDX 005).

18. HAMAND, J. Abortion—a way of life in Greece. *People*, **12**(3): 19–21 (1985).

19. DAVID, P. S. India. In: *Psychosocial aspects of abortion in Asia.* Nepal, Family Planning Association of Nepal, 1974.

20. MOROKVASIC, M. Sexuality and control of procreation. In: Young, K. et al., ed. *Of marriage and the market.* London, CSE Books, 1981, pp. 128–142.

21. DIGGORY, P. A review of abortion practices and their safety. In: Kierse, M. J. C. et al., ed. *Second trimester pregnancy termination.* Netherlands, Leiden University Press, 1982 (Boerhaave Series, Vol. 22).

22. COOK, R. J. & SENANAYKE, P., ed. *The human problem of abortion and legal dimensions.* London, International Planned Parenthood Federation, 1978.

23. HARRISON, P. On the septic ward. *People*, **4**(3): 12–13 (1977).

24. SHERRIS, J. D. & FOX, G. Infertility and sexually transmitted diseases. A public health challenge. *Population reports*, Series L, No. 4 (1983).

25. TIETZE, C. & BONGAATS, J. Fertility rates and abortion rates, simulations of family limitations. *Studies in family planning*, **6**: 114 (1975).

26. MOORE-CAVAR, E. C. *International inventory of information on induced abortion.* New York, Institute for the Study of Human Reproduction, 1974.

27. BHATIA, S. Traditional childbirth practices: implications for a rural maternal and child health program. *Studies in family planning*, **12**(2): 66–75 (1981).

28. SUN, T. H. ET AL. Trends in fertility, family size preference and family planning practice: Taiwan, 1961–76. *Studies in family planning*, **9**(4): 54–70 (1978).

29. LOVEL, H. & BAKOULA, C. Lack of family planning leading to induced abortion in rural Greece. *IPPF medical bulletin*, **19**(3): 1 (1985).

30. TIETZE, C. *Induced abortion. A world review.* 5th ed. New York, Population Council, 1983.

31. MACPHERSON, T. A. A retrospective study of maternal deaths in the Zimbabwean black. *Central African journal of medicine*, **27**(4): 57–60 (1981).

32. ARMON, P. J. Maternal deaths in the Kilimanjaro region of Tanzania. *Transactions of the Royal Society of Tropical Medicine and Hygiene*, **73**(3): 284–288 (1979).

# Chapter 7

# MATERNAL MORBIDITY

The figures for maternal mortality do not tell the full story of suffering caused by untreated complications in pregnancy and labour. Though exact figures are not known, it is thought that, for every woman who dies, about sixteen women suffer damage to their health which may last the rest of their lives. Some forms of maternal morbidity cause untold misery to individual women and their families, yet in many places ill health associated with childbearing is so common that people tend to accept it as normal and mostly unavoidable, no matter how severe.

## Morbidity in the period immediately after childbirth

The range of things that can go wrong during the puerperium (which, by convention, covers the first six weeks after childbirth or abortion) is very wide. Some disorders during this period are the result of complications that occur only during pregnancy and childbirth. Others are not specific to pregnancy, although their outcome may be affected by pregnancy. Yet others are direct results of traditional cultural practices.

Conditions specifically associated with the immediate post-delivery period include puerperal hypertension, peripartal cardiac failure, acute prolapse of the cervix and puerperal psychiatric illness.

### Puerperal hypertension

Sometimes women who have not previously had high blood pressure develop the condition following delivery. Alternatively, hypertension in the post-delivery period may be associated with pre-eclampsia (see Chapter 5). Most women whose blood pressure rises after delivery have no symptoms; the condition is discovered only through routine checks. Not much is known about the cause of this condition. The risks of developing it are least in women aged between 15 and 29 years, and highest in those younger or older than this, and those of high parity (1). Furthermore, it appears that black women are more susceptible than other races. Evidence suggests that in most cases of puerperal hypertension, the blood pressure gradually returns to normal. However, in a minority of women, the condition recurs during subsequent pregnancies and deliveries, and occasional deaths from complications such as heart failure and brain haemorrhage have been reported.

## Peripartal cardiac failure

For reasons which are not clearly understood, some women go into heart failure after delivery. Chest pain, intense shortness of breath, cough and swelling of the body, especially the feet and legs, are the predominant symptoms; there may also be other symptoms related to the presence of infection somewhere in the body. High blood pressure is a not uncommon finding in women with this kind of heart failure.

This bizarre complication of childbirth has been reported from practically every continent (1). Black women and women from the Republic of Korea appear to be particularly susceptible, but nowhere is the disease as common as among the Hausas of northern Nigeria. Researchers believe that it occurs in 1% of Hausa deliveries in the Zaria area of Nigeria, for example, and there is reason to suspect that certain cultural habits may play an important part (1). The following is a description of the traditional practice among women during the puerperium:

> For forty days or more after delivery, the traditional Hausa mother does not leave her compound, and lies twice daily for hours on a baked mud bed over a fire, which makes her very hot, splashes herself with scalding water, and eats highly spiced food, and a pap laced with *Kanwa*, a dried lake-salt.

Older women, those of high parity, and women with multiple pregnancies are most prone to peripartal cardiac failure. In Nigerian women the response to treatment is generally good. Approximately one-fifth of the patients with this condition suffer a recurrence which is identical to the initial episode, and although treatment for a prolonged period helps, it does not entirely eliminate the risk.

## Acute prolapse of the cervix

Women in labour should not be encouraged to bear down until the cervical canal is completely and fully dilated, so that the whole of the genital tract, from the uterus to the vulva, has become one continuous "tube". All trained birth attendants know this. However, in certain cultures traditional birth attendants are not aware of the normal changes in the cervix during labour, and women under their care are encouraged to bear down before they should, sometimes for hours or even days before conditions are ripe for the expulsion of the baby through the birth canal. As a result, the supports of the cervix become damaged and weak. The cervix may descend from its normal position high in the vagina, to the introitus and even beyond. When this happens, the whole of the cervix becomes swollen, sometimes reaching the size of two fists combined, and with the canal in it still closed. The swelling may also involve the vulva. Normal vaginal delivery becomes impossible and infection of the rest of the birth canal inevitably follows.

Reports describe the practice of encouraging women in labour to bear down too early among southern African peoples such as the Xhosa, Zulu and Pondo (2) and among women in Malawi.[1]

## Psychiatric illness in the puerperium

While organic illness accounts for most of the complications reported in pregnancy, childbirth and the puerperium, psychiatric illnesses also occur. Psychiatric illness may take one of several forms, which include neurotic reaction, states of confusion, affective disorders and schizophrenia. In most cases such disorders become manifest within the first week following childbirth. Infections, including puerperal sepsis, can trigger off psychiatric disturbance, and treatment should be directed towards the abnormal behaviour as well as towards any organic disease that may be present (3). Most women respond quite well to treatment, but a few may suffer relapse during subsequent childbirth and for years afterwards. During the early days of the puerperium there is a danger that the woman with a psychiatric disorder may cause serious harm to herself and to her own or to other women's babies. Infanticide and even suicide have been known to occur.

## Long-term sequelae of childbirth complications

The majority of long-term effects of childbearing under adverse conditions are related to obstructed labour, obstetric

---

[1] Bullough, C. H. W. *Traditional birth attendants in Malawi.* Thesis, Glasgow University, 1980.

haemorrhage and puerperal infection, with injuries from obstructed labour top of the list. Long-term problems include fistula, Sheehan's syndrome, pelvic inflammatory disease (PID), secondary infertility, ectopic pregnancy, anaemia, and uterovaginal prolapse.

## Fistula

During obstructed labour due to cephalopelvic disproportion, the fit of the baby's head in the mother's pelvis becomes very tight, making the soft tissue of the vagina and nearby structures vulnerable to serious injury. The uterus may rupture, with dire consequences (see Chapter 5), or a false passage may be created between the vagina and the urinary bladder; this is known as a vesicovaginal fistula. In about 50% of cases the fistula is over 2 cm in diameter, and in 10–15% the urethra is totally destroyed (4). The woman suffering from vesicovaginal fistula is unable to control her bladder, and leaks urine constantly through the vagina, wetting her thighs and legs. Injuries may also involve the rectum, in which case a rectovaginal fistula is formed, so that the vagina and thighs are soiled with leaking faeces. Reports from many places show that between 10% and 15% of women suffering from vesicovaginal fistula also have rectovaginal fistula (5). In time the skin of the vulva and thighs, being constantly soaked, becomes intolerably itchy.

For the individual sufferer, the social and psychological consequences of fistula can be staggering. Because of their incontinence, women with this condition have a highly offensive body odour, and as sympathy for their problems wears thin with time, they find themselves shunned by society. They are also likely to be childless, not only because they are rejected by their husbands, but also because any child they bear is likely to die at birth from prolonged obstructed labour. In a society where a woman's status depends on her fertility this carries an added stigma. In some societies fistula is thought to be the consequence of infidelity or wrong-doing. Many sufferers are divorced by their husbands and left to destitution.

Gynaecological surgery offers the only hope of restoring normal bladder and bowel function. Sometimes the operation is successful first time. However, not infrequently, repeated operations over a period of several years are necessary. Even so, some patients never recover their bladder function and remain permanently incontinent. Studies suggest that, as social outcasts, fistula sufferers often receive little support from husband or family when they seek treatment. Usually they live far away from hospitals with surgical facilities and are not aware of the fact that their condition is treatable. However, a study from Nigeria showed clearly that once aware of the possibility, such women are single-minded in their pursuit of treatment, selling their valued family possessions to raise the money for transport and treatment (6). In the final analysis, however, prevention provides the only satisfactory solution to the problem.

The majority of reports concerning fistula come from Africa. The condition is most common where women are prone to contracted pelvises and where early marriage and childbearing are the custom. The tragedy is that a high proportion of sufferers appear to be girls still in their teens. A report from Niger, for example, reveals that 80% of fistula patients were girls aged 15–19 (7), whereas 18% of a sample of fistula patients in Sudan were under 19 years old (8), and 33% of a sample in Nigeria were below 16 years (6).

Reports from the late 1950s to the 1970s indicate that each year individual gynaecologists from India (9), Pakistan (10), South Africa (11), western Nigeria (12), and Sudan (8) were treating between 20 and 80 fistula patients, who accounted for 2–16% of all major gynaecological operations. And in northern Nigeria in the 1970s, around 300 women a year with obstetric fistula were reporting for treatment to one team of specialists (see also Table 7.1). Today in northern Nigeria as many as 600 women are reported to be waiting for fistula repair, and some will wait in vain because of the pressure on the health services (13). A report from Ethiopia revealed that 30% of all gynaecological admissions to one hospital were for fistula repair (14). In Addis Ababa a 40-bed hospital has been devoted entirely to this operation since 1975.

## Neurological dysfunction

Prolonged obstructed labour may also cause injury to the nerves that cross the pelvic girdle, either from stretching or from pressure of the fetal head. The results of such injury include loss of sensation in parts of the skin of the feet, wasting of muscles in the legs and feet, and "drop foot". The worst-affected women become crippled for life and unable to walk except with crutches.

Table 7.1.  Major gynaecological operations at the
Ahmadu Bello University Hospital,
Zaria, Nigeria, 1970–1972

| Operation | Number |
|---|---|
| Vesicovaginal or rectovaginal fistula | |
| Vagina repair | 583 |
| Abdominal closure | 8 |
| Ureterocolic anastomosis | 23 |
| Pelvic floor repair | 146 |
| Ectopic gestation | 124 |
| Abdominal hysterectomy | |
| Wertheim's | 10 |
| Others | 51 |
| Laparotomy for pelvic inflammatory disease | 45 |
| Operation for benign ovarian tumour | 43 |
| Vaginal hysterectomy and pelvic floor repair | 35 |
| Myomectomy | 28 |
| Tubal ligation | 16 |
| Others | 18 |
| Total | 1130 |

*Source*: K. A. Harrison, personal communication, 1986.

Neurological dysfunction and fistula are often seen together
in the same woman. In a report from Nigeria, for instance,
17 women of a total of 65 with vesicovaginal fistula also had
obstetric palsy. Obstructed labour is the underlying cause of
both conditions. However, women who suffer from nerve
palsy and who do not have fistula tend to report early
enough for treatment to avoid long-term disability, whereas
women with fistula are shunned by their families and thus
slow to seek help.

## Vaginal stenosis

Wherever fistula has occurred during delivery there will be
damage to the vagina also. Over a period of time the injured
areas are replaced by dense scar tissue, and the vagina
becomes short, narrow and extremely rigid. Sometimes it can
barely admit a finger. This is vaginal stenosis, and it may
also be caused by puerperal or post-abortion infection, sometimes as a result of traditional practices. For example, the
practice of inserting caustic pessaries (see page 143) causes
intense local inflammation. As the inflammation subsides,
scars form along the wall of the vagina; these can be either
soft—in which case they do not often pose much of a problem—or very dense indeed, so that the vagina is distorted,
and the space in it becomes partially or totally occluded.

Vaginal injury of this nature affects menstruation, sexual intercourse and future childbearing. Intercourse becomes painful or indeed impossible in some cases; menstrual blood, unable to flow freely, gets trapped above the vagina, causing severe abdominal pain, and some women with vaginal stenosis can eventually no longer pass urine.

Treatment, where it involves more than manual dilatation of the vagina, may be very costly indeed, since it may require a series of highly skilled surgical operations to restore the vagina to normal.

The traditional practice of inserting caustic pessaries or other substances into the vagina is done for several reasons. One is to induce abortion, and some of the active ingredients reported are potassium permanganate in Côte d'Ivoire and Senegal (15), and crude potash in Ibadan, Nigeria (16). Another reason is to expedite delivery where labour has become prolonged and obstructed. For this particular purpose leaves and various oils are commonly used, although mixtures containing mud and cow dung are also reported. Among some East African people, for instance, cow dung is packed into the woman's vagina if labour is prolonged.[1] Sometimes, substances are inserted into the vagina to cause it to shrink after childbirth (17), presumably for the husband's pleasure. The use of salt, for example, is relatively common in some Eastern Mediterranean countries, but is reported to be on the wane. Not long ago in Kuwait, salt-induced vaginal stenosis after delivery was found in as many as 16 women per 1000 deliveries (18).

## Sheehan's syndrome

Sheehan's syndrome is a long-term problem associated with obstetric haemorrhage and concerns the pituitary gland. This important gland, the size of a pea, lies protected within a small socket at the base of the skull. Its importance lies in the fact that it is the leading endocrine gland, producing hormones that control the activities of other endocrine glands such as the thyroid, ovaries, and suprarenal glands.

When shock follows severe obstetric haemorrhage, adjustments in the circulation aimed at combating the effects are brought into play automatically by the body. Blood is diverted to organs, such as the heart and brain, whose

---

[1] *Traditional birth practices.* Unpublished document WHO/MCH/85.11.

function is absolutely essential for survival. The pituitary gland is one of the organs adversely affected under these circumstances. Its blood supply is markedly reduced, resulting in the death of portions of the gland and a fall in the amount of some of the hormones that it produces. The resultant loss of function depends on the extent of damage to the pituitary gland, but it may be profound. Lactation ceases, as does menstruation, and a host of other complaints may follow. These include dizziness, muscle and joint pains, general weakness, constipation, anaemia, intolerance to cool weather, episodes of unconsciousness, loss of pubic and axillary hair, and depigmentation of the skin. Premature aging with shrinkage of the genital organs is another important feature of this disease, and in advanced cases there may be marked curvature of the spine.

Notwithstanding these symptoms, many sufferers go unrecognized for years. Treatment of patients with Sheehan's syndrome involves replacement of some of the hormones that are no longer produced naturally. But in developing countries, these are practically never available, and when they are, the cost may be prohibitive. The prevention of Sheehan's syndrome is therefore very important, and this depends squarely on blood being available for transfusion, and being used effectively to prevent shock from obstetric haemorrhage (*12*). (Interestingly, pituitary necrosis does not appear to follow shock from any other type of haemorrhage).

It is not known exactly how frequently Sheehan's syndrome occurs. Rough estimates of its incidence range from 1.7% to 14% of cases of postpartum haemorrhage (*14*). Reports since 1964 have mostly been from Africa, particularly Algeria, Senegal, Tunisia and Zimbabwe (*19–21*).

## Chronic pelvic inflammatory disease (PID)

In cases of puerperal sepsis the infection is often not confined to the uterus. In the absence of effective treatment, it may spread through the genital tract, sometimes causing damage to the fallopian tubes and ovaries. Scars that form around the uterus as a result of infection may cause it to change position, adding to the wide range of symptoms experienced by the affected woman. Pain is the dominant symptom, and in severe cases of PID it occurs during defecation, when passing urine, during sexual intercourse, and at and around menstruation. Low backache is common and the menstrual periods become irregular and very heavy. Widespread damage to the reproductive system caused by chronic PID often leads to permanent infertility, and the pain and discomfort affect the daily lives of sufferers.

Treatment with pain-relieving drugs and antibiotics never completely cures chronic PID, and in the end radical surgery—that is, removal of the uterus and the fallopian tubes—is often necessary. This procedure does eventually relieve the pain, but the resulting loss of menstruation and fertility tends to bring its own brand of misery.

Chronic PID can also lead to problems of another kind. Years after the episode of puerperal sepsis, women with chronic PID may develop gynaecological disorders, such as uterine fibroids, uterovaginal prolapse, and ovarian diseases, which require surgery. In such women, most of the organs in the abdomen tend to be stuck firmly together because of the scars that formed around them following puerperal sepsis. Thus the separation of these organs during surgery in order to remove those that are diseased becomes very difficult, and in the process the intestines, bladder and other structures may be injured.

## Infertility

It is apparent from the previous descriptions of health problems associated with pregnancy and labour that a number of conditions can lead to infertility. The most common cause of infertility in many developing countries is blockage in, or damage to, the fallopian tubes (see Table 7.2).

Table 7.2. Prevalence of fallopian tube damage in women attending clinics for treatment of infertility

| Clinic location | Number of women | % with tubal abnormalities |
| --- | --- | --- |
| Nairobi, Kenya | 104 | 73 |
| Libreville, Gabon | 228 | 44 |
| Kef, Tunisia | 114 | 56 |
| Highlands, Papua New Guinea | 220 | 86 |
| North Sulawesi Peninsula, Indonesia | 634 | 62 |

Source: Sherris & Fox (22).

Though PID associated with puerperal infection is a common cause of tubal damage, sexually transmitted diseases can have the same effect, and reports of tubal infertility often do not distinguish between the two. However, where rates of secondary infertility (failure to conceive again after a previous pregnancy) are high, this may indicate that the complications of pregnancy and labour have played a major role. In Cameroon, for instance, a study of women aged 15–50 in different regions of the country revealed that between 3% and 17% suffered from primary infertility, while the rates for secondary infertility ranged from 14% to 39% (22).

## Ectopic pregnancy

An ectopic pregnancy is one where the fertilized ovum develops outside the uterus. The fallopian tube is by far the commonest site for ectopic pregnancy, and damage to this organ following infection is the underlying cause (see Chapter 5). Since untreated puerperal infection and sexually transmitted diseases frequently cause damage to fallopian tubes, ectopic pregnancy is particularly common in places where PID is rife. In fact it has been estimated that the chance of ectopic pregnancy is seven times higher than normal for a woman who has suffered pelvic infection (34).

Estimates of the frequency of ectopic pregnancy have been given as 36 per 1000 births in Jamaica (23), as 1 per 4.3 deliveries in a hospital in Benin City, Nigeria, with 63% of cases exhibiting gross signs of PID (24), and as 1 for every 9 major gynaecological operations in Zaria, Nigeria (see Table 7.1). In Kampala, Uganda, 2 out of every 5 women admitted with major gynaecological disease had either PID or ectopic pregnancy, according to one report (25).

## Anaemia

For a number of reasons (see Chapters 4 and 5), anaemia is common among women in developing countries. Pregnancy and childbirth can exacerbate the condition, either through loss of blood or through failure to meet the extra requirements for iron and folic acid during pregnancy with an adequate diet or with special supplements of these nutrients. Not surprisingly, anaemia in non-pregnant women is a major health problem throughout the Third World. In one extensive review, practically all the women in some populations had haemoglobin concentrations below normal levels compared with a mere 4–7% of women in the developed countries studied (26).

The danger of severe anaemia in pregnancy is well recognized (see Chapter 5). Only comparatively recently have the serious and far-reaching effects of anaemia in the non-pregnant population been fully realized. These are well illustrated by the results of a study in Sri Lanka in which the productivity of moderately anaemic and non-anaemic female plantation workers was compared (27). The average weight of tea picked per day by the anaemic group was found to be considerably less than that of the non-anaemic group. After anaemia had been corrected by iron supplements, work output rose to levels comparable to those of the women who were not anaemic. Even in purely economic terms the implications of these results are serious, especially in societies where women are largely responsible for food production.

## Uterovaginal prolapse

Uterovaginal prolapse is another possible consequence of childbirth among women who are poorly nourished, are overburdened with hard physical work, have many babies, and have little chance of professional care during pregnancy and labour. It was described earlier how, during unsupervised deliveries, the supports of the cervix and vagina can be injured. If recovery is incomplete, as is often the case, the cervix, carrying with it the uterus and the vagina, may protrude outside the vulval opening. In such cases the descent of the vagina affects the urinary bladder (cystocele) and also the rectum and anus (rectocele).

Uterovaginal prolapse causes much local discomfort and also affects the passing of urine and other bodily functions. The affected woman is sometimes unable to control her bladder and may leak urine when coughing, sneezing or even dancing (stress incontinence); alternatively, the prolapsed uterus may partially block urination. There may be constipation and constant low backache. The cervix, if displaced permanently outside the introitus, ulcerates, bleeds and becomes infected, exuding a foul-smelling discharge. Many women with prolapse are in their thirties, and the presence of prolapse affects subsequent pregnancies. The risk of both spontaneous abortion and premature labour increases (28). Large uterovaginal prolapse sometimes co-exists with pregnancy, and a report from India shows how this is associated with traumatic delivery, heavy loss of fetal lives, and puerperal sepsis afterwards (29).

A survey of the health status of women in nine countries
(*30*) revealed that many sufferers do not recognize the
condition as abnormal (see Table 7.3). Few of the women in
the survey complained of the disease although on examination between 2% and 28% of them were found to be suffering from it. There were similar findings in Brazil, where
uterovaginal prolapse was discovered in 4% of women
reporting to hospital for non-gynaecological complaints (*35*).

Considering the circumstances leading to uterovaginal
prolapse, it is not surprising that women of high parity and
advanced age are more often affected than the young and
those of lesser parity.

Table 7.3.  Prolapse and parity

| Country and group | Percentage of women with uterovaginal prolapse at parity: | | | | | |
|---|---|---|---|---|---|---|
| | 0 | 1 and 2 | 3 and 4 | 5 and 6 | 7+ | All parities |
| Colombia | | | | | | |
| Old urban zone | 0 | 5 | 13 | 27 | 38 | 19 |
| Newly settled | 3 | 2 | 8 | 17 | 25 | 8 |
| India (Ganhigram) | | | | | | |
| Muslim | 2 | 2 | 2 | 2 | 3 | 2 |
| Scheduled castes | 0 | 0 | 2 | 6 | 0 | 2 |
| Upper caste | 0 | 1 | 3 | 2 | 9 | 2 |
| Other Hindus | 0 | 1 | 2 | 5 | 1 | 2 |
| Islamic Republic of Iran (Teheran) | | | | | | |
| Muslim | 1 | 12 | 21 | 28 | 11 | 9 |
| Armenian | 1 | 3 | 5 | 7 | 1 | 2 |
| Lebanon (Beirut) | | | | | | |
| Shiites | 5 | 6 | 18 | 32 | 40 | 26 |
| Maronites | 0 | 8 | 28 | 38 | 46 | 28 |
| Pakistan | | | | | | |
| Urban | 1 | 6 | 11 | 16 | 14 | 11 |
| Semiurban | 0 | 12 | 22 | 26 | 37 | 25 |
| Philippines (Manila) | | | | | | |
| Rural | 0 | 2 | 4 | 8 | 15 | 6 |
| Urban | 12 | 4 | 10 | 12 | 15 | 9 |
| Syrian Arab Republic | | | | | | |
| Damascus | 0 | 5 | 10 | 11 | 13 | 10 |
| Sweida | 0 | 1 | 2 | 3 | 7 | 3 |
| Rural Aleppo | 1 | 6 | 6 | 9 | 10 | 8 |
| Turkey (Ankara) | | | | | | |
| Rural | – | 2 | 3 | —3— | | 3 |
| Semiurban | 0 | 3 | 3 | —6— | | 4 |

*Source*: Omran & Standley (*30*).

# Health problems associated with traditional surgical practices

## Female circumcision

Of all the traditional surgical practices that can lead to morbidity, the best known is probably female circumcision—an operation in which part or all of the external genitalia of a woman are cut away. In the most extreme form, infibulation, the two sides of the vulva are subsequently stitched together to leave a very small opening. The practice is reported from parts of Egypt, Ethiopia, Kenya, Somalia and Sudan (31). The exact incidence is not known, but it is estimated that between 30 million and 74 million women have undergone this traditional operation (32). Though female circumcision is not a health consequence of pregnancy and childbirth, it deserves mention here because it can have a profound effect on the outcome of pregnancy. By distorting the introitus and muscle tone through scarring, the radical forms of female circumcision cause difficulties and often intense distress during sexual intercourse, and obstruction at the time of delivery.

## Gishiri cut

The word "gishiri" means salt in Hausa. But it also refers to a traditional surgical procedure in which the vagina is cut, usually with a razor blade (33). As far as can be ascertained, the practice is found only among the Hausa people of West Africa, particularly in northern Nigeria. Gishiri cuts are most commonly performed during prolonged obstructed labour in the mistaken belief that this operation will relieve the obstruction. Other conditions known to have been "treated" by gishiri cut include menstrual disturbances, marital problems, infertility, backache, dysuria, headaches and even goitre. In one extreme case of a very young teenage bride, "the husband himself had used a razor blade to cut his wife, in order to widen her introitus for intercourse" (6).

Cuts in the anterior wall of the vagina are most common. In most cases they are small and the bleeding which follows soon ceases. Where deeper cuts are made, however, the urinary bladder and urethra may be completely divided, causing urinary fistula; the fetus may be injured in the case of a woman in labour, and death of the mother from the ensuing haemorrhage and infection is not unknown (6).

The practice still continues, though almost exclusively among women with no formal education who are most bound by tradition. In a report on vesicovaginal fistula in 1443 women in Zaria, northern Nigeria, gishiri cut was thought to be directly responsible in 13% of the women (6).

## Conclusion

Ill health associated with childbearing is so common in developing countries that many people have developed a fatalistic attitude towards it. The scale of suffering is therefore probably far greater than is generally supposed. Most of this suffering is needless, for we have the knowledge to avoid many of the problems that cause it. Chronic PID, ectopic pregnancy, fistula and its associated problems of stenosis and obstetric paralysis, uterovaginal prolapse, and the consequences of obstetric haemorrhage can be prevented if women are given proper care during pregnancy, childbirth and the puerperium. However, the suffering caused by traditional practices such as female circumcision, gishiri cut, and the use of harmful substances in the vagina will not cease until attitudes towards women change and the deeply rooted cultural habits that are so dangerous to their health are abandoned.

## References

1. DAVIDSON, N. McD. & PARRY, E. H. O. Peri-partum cardiac failure. *Quarterly journal of medicine*, New Series, XLVII (*188*): 431–461 (1978).

2. BAGNELL, D. Obstetric rituals and taboos. *Nursing times*, 18 July: 1130–1133 (1974).

3. EBIE, J. C. Psychiatric illness in the puerperium among Nigerians. *Tropical and geographical medicine*, **24**: 253–256 (1972).

4. BARNAUD, P. L'obstétrique outre-mer: introduction. *Médecine tropicale*, **43**(1): 9–11 (1983).

5. PERQUIS, P. Fistules vesico-vaginales obstétricales en Afrique noire. *Médecine tropicale*, **31**(5): 1–9 (1979).

6. TAHZIB, F. Vesicovaginal fistula in Nigerian children. *Lancet*, **2** (8467): 1291–1293 (1985).

7. DOCQUIER, J. & SAKO, A. Fistules recto-vaginales d'origine obstétricale. *Médecine d'Afrique noire*, **30**(5): 213–215 (1983).

8. MUSTAFA, A. Z. & RUSHWAN, H. M. E. Acquired genito-urinary fistula in the Sudan. *Journal of obstetrics and gynaecology of the British Commonwealth*, **78**: 1039–1043 (1971).

9. NAIDU, P. M. Vesico-vaginal fistulae: an experience with 208

cases. *Journal of obstetrics and gynaecology of the British Commonwealth,* **69**: 311 (1962).

10. Azis, S. A. Urinary fistulae from obstetrical trauma. *Journal of obstetrics and gynaecology of the British Commonwealth,* **72**: 765–768 (1965).

11. Coetzee, T. & Lithgow, D. M. Obstetric fistulae of the urinary tract. *Journal of obstetrics and gynaecology of the British Commonwealth,* **73**: 837–844 (1966).

12. Lawson, J. B. Birth-canal injuries. *Proceedings of the Royal Society of Medicine,* **61**: 368–370 (1968).

13. Lister, U. G. Vesico-vaginal fistulae. *Postgraduate doctor,* **6**(10): 321–323 (1984).

14. Habte-Gabr, E. et al. Analysis of admissions to Gondar Hospital in north-western Ethiopia, 1971–1972. *Ethiopian medical journal,* **14**: 49–59 (1976).

15. Sangaret, M. & Bohoussou, K. Les lésions vaginales par le permanganate de potassium. *Afrique médicale,* **13**(20): 403–408 (1974).

16. Lawson, J. B. The management of genitourinary fistulae. *Clinical obstetrics and gynaecology,* **5**(1): 209–236 (1978).

17. Abu-Lughod, M. Obstetrical aspects of salt-induced vaginal and cervical atresia. *Journal of the Kuwait Medical Association,* **3**: 145–149 (1969).

18. Fahmy, K. Necrotic obstetric vesico-vaginal fistulae. *Journal of the Kuwait Medical Association,* **6**(3): 167–176 (1972).

19. Dano, P. et al. Le syndrome de Sheehan (à propos de 5 cas chez l'Afrique). *Dakar médicale,* **27**(3): 323–330 (1982).

20. Sankale, M. et al. Le syndrome de Sheehan en Afrique noire (à propos de neuf cas, dont cinq personnels). *African journal of medicine and medical science,* **7**: 65–69 (1978).

21. Chimbira, T. H. K. & Kasule, J. Amenorrhoea in Zimbabwean women. *Journal of obstetrics and gynaecology of East Africa,* **3**: 131–134 (1984).

22. Sherris, J. D. & Fox, G. Infertility and sexually transmitted diseases. A public health challenge. *Population reports,* Series L, No. 4 (1983).

23. Douglas, C. P. Tubal ectopic pregnancy. *British medical journal,* **2**: 838–841 (1963).

24. Oronsaye, A. U. & Odiase, G. I. Incidence of ectopic pregnancy in Benin City, Nigeria. *Tropical doctor,* **11**(4): 160–163 (1981).

25. Trussel, R. R. Pelvic inflammatory disease. *Proceedings of the Royal Society of Medicine,* **61**: 365–368 (1968).

26. Royston, E. The prevalence of nutritional anaemia in women in developing countries: a critical review of available information. *World health statistics quarterly,* **35**: 52–91 (1982).

27. Edgerton, V. R. et al. Iron-deficiency anaemia and its effect on worker productivity and activity patterns. *British medical journal,* **2**: 1546–1549 (1979).

28. Lavery, J. P. & Boey, C. S. Uterine prolapse with pregnancy. *Obstetrics and gynaecology*, **42**(5): 681–683 (1973).

29. Das, R. K. Genital prolapse in pregnancy and labor. *International surgery*, **56**: 260–266 (1971).

30. Omran, A. R. & Standley, C. C. *Family formation patterns and health.* Vol. 1 and 2. Geneva, World Health Organization, 1976 and 1978.

31. Cook, R. Damage to physical health from pharaonic circumcision (infibulation) of females. In: *Traditional practices affecting the health of women and children.* Alexandria, WHO Regional Office for the Eastern Mediterranean, 1979 (WHO/EMRO Technical Publication No. 2), pp. 53–69.

32. United Nations Economic and Social Council. *Report of the working group on traditional practices affecting the health of women and children. Commission of Human Rights, 3 February–14 March 1986.* Paris, 1986.

33. Trevitt, L. Attitudes and customs among the Hausa in Zaria City. *Savanna*, **2**: 223–226 (1973).

34. Westrom, L. Incidence, prevalence and trends of acute pelvic inflammatory disease and its consequences in industrialized countries. *American journal of obstetrics and gynaecology*, **38**(7): 880 (1980).

35. Pinotti, J. A. et al. Preventative obstetrics and gynecology program: pilot plan for integrated medical care. *Bulletin of the Pan American Health Organization*, **15**(2): 104–112 .(1981).

# Chapter 8

# THE ROLE OF THE HEALTH SERVICES IN PREVENTING MATERNAL DEATHS

We know already how to prevent most of the common end causes of maternal death, such as eclampsia, obstructed labour, haemorrhage, or sepsis. The fact that these have become rarities in the industrialised world, in some developing countries and in all but some rural areas of China, proves conclusively that we know enough to act effectively now (1).

Maternal death has many causes, and it therefore requires action on several fronts simultaneously to combat it. The need for improvement in the social status of women, to ensure that they receive the same care and attention as boys as they grow up, and give them wider horizons as adults, and recognition of their daily labour, has been discussed at length in an earlier chapter. This chapter describes the role of the health services—both directly and indirectly—in preventing maternal death and ill health.

Of the interventions described, some yield quick and obvious results, while others affect childbearing in the longer term. However, they should not be seen as separate and alternative approaches to saving lives, but as parts of a whole, all dependent upon and reinforcing each other. Naturally, the relative importance of each intervention will depend on the circumstances and health problems of each particular place.

The interventions are described from the point of view of the woman's needs at different stages, and they follow a sequence which runs from the years preceding pregnancy, through the prenatal period and childbirth itself, to the puerperium. Family planning is also included, since every maternal health care system should have family planning as one of its essential components (see Chapter 9).

## Health care before pregnancy

Some of the major problems of pregnancy and childbirth—such as cephalopelvic disproportion and anaemia—may have their roots in the mother's own childhood (see Chapter 4).

Prevention of these problems therefore needs to begin many years before pregnancy with, for instance, better nutrition for girls, and more attention to their health in early childhood, including making sure that they are appropriately immunized.

Since these are largely questions of how parents bring up their children and the priority they give to the needs of sons or daughters, the role of the health sector at this stage is largely supportive and educational.

However, there are ways in which the health services can identify the problem of discrimination against female children, and take active measures to combat its ill effects. Higher mortality rates for female infants than for males are a crucial indicator of serious discrimination against girls, especially since females have a biological advantage that should, under normal circumstances, bias infant mortality rates in their favour.

Where civil registration is poor or non-existent, these data may not be available, in which case the keeping of sex-specific clinic or immunization records can be used to alert the health services to discrimination against female children.

Whatever the means used to identify it, when discrimination is known to exist, the health services can play an active role in combating it by such measures as setting specific targets for female coverage in nutrition or immunization pro-grammes, or perhaps giving incentives, such as concessional rates (where charges exist) for health care. In societies where sex discrimination is deep-rooted, however, it is often necessary in the first place to create awareness among health and social workers of the risks run by female children so that they realize that there is a need to pay special attention to them.

There are other aspects of development which, though not primarily the responsibility of the health sector, contribute to maternal health by increasing the chances that women will be in good general health before they start having children. Among these are the provision of sanitation and safe water supplies, which not only save time and energy for women in fetching water, often from far away, but also cut down on the transmission of some communicable diseases, such as viral hepatitis and hookworm. Development programmes involving food production and processing, for personal consumption or to generate income, also have the potential to enhance women's nutritional status, provided the benefits of their labours are not diverted to other family members or anyone else.

## Health education

Well designed health education, both in the school setting and in the community, can do a great deal in the prevention of maternal ill health. Among the messages that need to be communicated concerning reproductive health is the danger of very early marriage and adolescent pregnancy. Other appropriate subjects are the advantages of spacing pregnancies and the reasons that prenatal care is necessary.

Ideally, reproductive health topics, including contraception, should be part of health education in schools, though this is not always easy to achieve. Where strong cultural or religious beliefs prohibit the free discussion of sexual matters— particularly with young unmarried people—health educators are likely to be faced with a dilemma.

At the community level also, education that promotes values contrary to those of the people will meet with resistance, so sensitivity to the prevailing attitudes and beliefs is always essential. Furthermore, health education should be participatory—allowing for a genuine two-way exchange of ideas- -because it is as important for those who provide health care to understand and respect the "health culture" of the people as it is for members of the community to learn new ways of safeguarding their own health.

Some education projects have used particularly innovative methods to achieve this dynamic process. Puppets have been used in Nigeria to deliver health messages and stimulate discussion, while in Malawi, recently, some performing arts students from the university established a theatre group in cooperation with the primary health care staff to visit communities (2). Initially, some members of the university theatre group together with primary health care staff visited the community to discuss local health problems with their representatives. Sketches were then devised to illustrate these, which involved the audience first in discussion and gradually as participants in the drama. The drama was particularly effective in breaking down traditional inhibitions, and from the sketches various solutions to the problems emerged. A measure of the pilot project's success was the fact that a group of women led by a traditional birth attendant, without any assistance from the theatre group, subsequently devised a sketch to articulate the particular problems of women in the community.

Advances in communications technology have put many other tools at the disposal of educators today. Films and videos are taken into villages and urban communities by health education units, and many make good use of the mass media to get their messages across to people.

However, these things do not happen in a vacuum. Health education demands real commitment. It takes time, energy and resources and cannot simply be added on to a busy working schedule. Commitment should start at the top with policy-makers, and health personnel at all levels of the service should be encouraged to practise it.

But health education need not be the exclusive domain of health personnel. Among others, community development workers, agriculturalists, and teachers of many disciplines can all be made more aware of health issues—perhaps by doctors giving guest talks at training colleges, etc.—and encouraged to discuss them during the course of their work.

## Traditional practices

There is a large variety of traditional practices that affect the health of women, some of which are of benefit, some of which are neutral in effect, and some of which are harmful. The role of the health services in respect of such practices is to support those that are positive, respect those that are neutral, and replace or abolish those that are negative.

Among the traditional practices that are of positive benefit are some that encourage delivery of babies with the mother in the upright position, perhaps on a "birthing stool", rather than supine; or that encourage the suckling of the baby immediately after delivery, thus stimulating uterine contractions, which encourage the expulsion of the placenta.

In the opinion of one obstetrician (3), "A significant number [of traditional practices] need to be infiltrated into modern obstetrics. These include giving emotional and physical support to the woman, allowing her to remain physically in control of labour, and to remain a person rather than merely a birth canal navigated by strangers who remove the child just when it should be in her arms and who design rituals for the convenience of the attendants and not of the woman."

Of the harmful traditional practices that affect women, female circumcision can have particularly serious consequences. Here, health personnel have an important educational role to play, though national or local women's organizations will play the major part in combating it. Besides information about the health consequences of female circumcision, the health sector can provide a forum where this extremely complex and sensitive issue can be discussed, as well as giving encouragement and support to those in the forefront of the campaign to abolish it.

## Family planning

Finally, a great contribution can be made to maternal health by easily available and acceptable contraceptives (see also Chapter 6). The avoidance of pregnancies at too young or too old an age, and the avoidance of pregnancies that are too closely spaced, or that are unwanted for any reason, would also reduce the total risk of mortality (see Chapter 9).

The provision of contraceptives through family planning programmes is the best way of avoiding unwanted pregnancies and subsequent abortion. However, even with good family planning services unwanted pregnancies still occur, and, recognizing the tragically high mortality rates associated with illicit abortion, some countries have legalized termination of pregnancy. The complex issues involved and their implications for the health services are explored in Chapter 6.

## Health care during pregnancy

### Prenatal care

Potentially, one of the most effective health interventions for the prevention of maternal mortality and morbidity is prenatal care, particularly in places where the general health status of women is very poor.

Prenatal care has several major functions:

(a) the promotion of health during pregnancy through advice and educational activities;

(b) the screening, identification, and referral if necessary of women with risk factors; and

(c) the monitoring of health throughout pregnancy in order to detect and deal with problems if and when they occur.

## Health promotion

Health education during prenatal care may be given either individually and informally or more systematically in groups. As well as covering such general topics as nutrition and self-care during pregnancy, the opportunity must be taken to inform women about the danger signs that all is not well with a pregnancy, and what action to take under the circumstances. These signs include:

(a) swelling of the feet, face, and hands;

(b) vaginal bleeding;

(c) early rupture of the membranes.

Other essential information to impart is the fact that any woman who has previously had a caesarean section must deliver in hospital, and that no woman must be in labour more than twelve hours without seeking medical help. (This interval of time should be explained in locally appropriate terms—not everyone can tell the time or possesses a watch). Sexual intercourse during the last month of pregnancy, as it relates to the risk of premature rupture of the membranes, may also be an appropriate subject for discussion. In addition, health education during prenatal care should address the post-delivery period—the care and nourishment of the future infant, breast-feeding and the advisability of birth spacing.

When it is done well, prenatal health education can help to build good relations between the mothers and the health services which will benefit the women and their families in the future as well.

## Screening

The main purpose of screening for risk factors is to detect those women who are more likely than others to have an adverse outcome of pregnancy, and to refer them to a more skilled and better-equipped level of care—both prenatally for more accurate assessment and later for safe management of potentially difficult labour. Screening must be a regular, not a one-time, procedure because women may develop risk factors late in pregnancy.

This type of prenatal care may be provided in health centres or aid posts, in mobile clinics, or in the outpatient departments of hospitals. (This is one of the few instances in which hospitals involve themselves in primary preventive care. This set-up is ideal for providing well supervised training in prenatal care, but, except in cities, hospital-based clinics are usually too far from people's homes to provide high coverage, and they are also unnecessarily expensive.)

Usually a list of risk factors is taught to the providers of prenatal health care, and this is likely to include such commonly recognized factors as: five or more previous deliveries; first pregnancy; age younger or older than optimum for childbearing; small stature; low weight at the beginning of pregnancy; history of previous instrumental delivery or fistula repair; history of other complications in a previous pregnancy, such as a hypertensive disorder or haemorrhage; the presence of a medical disorder that will be exacerbated by pregnancy, such as heart disease or diabetes mellitus; history of previous perinatal death. To these may be added some social risk factors of particular relevance locally, such as, for example, difficult home conditions, destitution, or very low intelligence. A simple list gives no clue to the relative importance of the risk factors—either singly or in combination—so criteria for referral also have to be established. These will vary from place to place, but care should always be taken to ensure that, as far as possible, women are not referred unnecessarily, thereby putting undue strain on health care facilities higher up the chain. Besides, if there are too many "false alarms", women will tend to disregard the advice of the prenatal staff. In practice, referral only works well when it is very selective.

When deciding how best to use risk factors for referral, two major points should be taken into consideration: how strong is the link between the risk factor and a bad outcome? And, how serious is the bad outcome? i.e., is the mother's life at risk?

If there is a very strong link between a risk factor and a potentially fatal outcome (e.g., where the mother has a contracted pelvis) then referral is essential. This is so, too, where a combination of "weak" risk factors adds up to a strong possibility that a woman will suffer complications during delivery. Because there are not usually many women with very serious risk factors, there is little danger of overloading the system by referring them automatically.

The same cannot be said, however, in the case of risk factors with a weaker link to a bad outcome, where there may be large numbers of women involved. Therefore, in deciding the referral criteria that will make optimum use of the health facilities without overloading the system, it is also necessary to know the prevalence of particular conditions. This may require some epidemiological research. Alternatively an informed guess about prevalence can be made based on similar situations elsewhere, and this can be adjusted in the light of experience.

Another point to be borne in mind when a referral system is being designed is the skill of the person who has to identify the risk and take the decision about referral. A health worker who has very limited training, and therefore limited skill in identifying risk factors and judging how serious an indication they are of future problems, will naturally need a different referral protocol from someone with deeper knowledge and better judgement.

Screening and referral can be very effective in saving lives, but for this to be so other links in the chain also need to be considered. There must, for example, be adequate transport for women referred to the next level of care, and this level must offer a larger range of services of higher quality than the referring unit. A weak link anywhere in the chain can render the whole system ineffective, as was well illustrated by a community study in a rural area of the Gambia with an extremely high maternal mortality rate. The study found that, as far as women at special risk were concerned, the possible benefits of prenatal care were diffused by an inadequate referral system: the only place where blood transfusion and obstetric services were available was the government hospital in the capital, Banjul, many miles and a boat trip away (4).

Before leaving the topic of risk screening, mention must be made of the value of home-based maternal record cards. Such a record could cover each pregnancy separately, but a maternal health record covering a number of years, and containing details of risk factors, the course and outcome of each pregnancy, and information concerning family planning care, is much better. Besides giving the mother herself, and her family, valuable information on which to act, records can make a substantial difference to the quality and effectiveness of prenatal care: nothing else is so likely to facilitate the flow of valuable information between primary level and referral level, between health centre and hospital.

## Health monitoring

Among the important monitoring functions of prenatal care are the detection and treatment, or prevention, of anaemia which everywhere plays a major role in maternal mortality and morbidity (see Chapter 5).

However, the measurement of haemoglobin for the detection of anaemia is frequently carried out very unsatisfactorily. It may be that the tests are not done at the health centre where prenatal care is given but that women are expected to go to a hospital probably some distance away. A woman may not go to the hospital for the test, or, if she does, the hospital may fail to pass the results back to the health centre. Procedural problems such as these need to be recognized and eliminated for prenatal care to be efficient in combating anaemia.

Malaria plays a significant role in anaemia in many parts of the developing world, besides which the effects of the disease are particularly severe during the first pregnancy and the risks of cerebral malaria and death are greatly increased. The increasing prevalence of chloroquine resistance in the malaria parasite has made the management of the disease in pregnancy ever more complex. The effect on the unborn child of the newer antimalarial drugs has not yet been established, so routine chemoprophylaxis for pregnant women in areas of chloroquine-resistant malaria cannot be recommended. In these areas, pregnant women must be closely monitored for fever, and treated promptly if malaria is suspected, because the complications of the disease itself are potentially more severe than the effects of therapy. In malarious areas where chloroquine resistance is not yet a problem, however, chemoprophylaxis can be instituted as a routine part of prenatal care.

Prenatal care has other important and potentially life-saving functions. One of these is the detection and management of pregnancy-induced hypertension (pre-eclampsia). This condition can be detected at an early stage by periodically measuring the blood pressure, examining for swelling of the tissues, especially pitting oedema of the lower leg, detecting any sudden increase in weight, or taking note of warning symptoms such as severe headaches. Midwives should be trained to carry out such monitoring, and traditional birth attendants should also be taught the danger signals and instructed to send any woman exhibiting them for appropriate examination and care. With rest, and drug treatment where necessary, the development of full-blown eclampsia can be prevented.

Another important function of prenatal care is the prompt referral to hospital of women who have vaginal bleeding. Many deaths from antepartum haemorrhage, whether due to partial detachment of the placenta or to placenta praevia, can be prevented if action is taken on the earliest warning sign. However, information about bleeding may need active prompting by health staff. In the case of placenta praevia such bleeding is generally painless, intermittent and ceases of its own accord, so women may not report it spontaneously.

Prenatal care should also include examination to determine the position of the fetus after the seventh month, in order to detect breech presentation or transverse lie, which would indicate the need for professional attendance during delivery. Staff carrying out the examination should also try to detect the presence of twins.

## Effectiveness of prenatal care

The reason that prenatal care is so important a component of maternal health care has been expressed succinctly by an obstetrician from Nigeria: "Today in developing countries, as was the case fifty years ago in the developed countries, a large proportion of the population is ill-housed, poorly nourished, in bad health, and largely ignorant of what is good for them and their babies. Until people prosper and economic benefits become widely spread, prenatal surveillance can provide the care needed to offset some of the harmful effects of large-scale poverty and underdevelopment" (K. A. Harrison, personal communication, 1986).

In support of this view it has been almost universally observed that the vast majority of deaths in childbirth occur among "unbooked cases", i.e., emergency admissions of women who have had no previous care whatever. For example, in a study in the north-west of Zaire, of 3413 women who attended a rural hospital between 1981 and 1983 for delivery of their babies, it was calculated that the risk of death was increased 15-fold for women who had not received prenatal care compared with those who had.[1] Similarly, a survey of maternal deaths in Addis Ababa found a rate of 2.4 per 1000 deliveries among women who had received prenatal care compared with a rate of 6.4 per 1000 for those who had had none (5).

Systematic studies showing that prenatal care in developing countries is effective are, however, scarce. One such study in Chile attempted to evaluate prenatal care by assessing the quality of care in different areas using a set of carefully considered indicators. It found that high rates of maternal and perinatal death correlated with low scores on quality of care, and vice versa (6).

So, too, assessment of prenatal care in Zaria, northern Nigeria, demonstrated that it was effective in saving lives, with some particularly interesting results among girls aged 15 years or younger (7). Those of this age group who sought prenatal care were given iron and folic acid supplements and malaria chemoprophylaxis, primarily to counteract anaemia. This treatment also had the effect of enhancing growth and physical development in the girls during their pregnancy, which was not the case with the girls who did not seek prenatal care or receive the treatment. Increase in height of the order of 8–16 cm between first attendance at the pre-natal clinic and delivery about 20 weeks later was observed, and this had the effect of cutting dramatically the incidence of cephalopelvic disproportion and obstructed labour.

The case for prenatal care is well made. However, there are some common problems that occur and that can undermine the effectiveness of care if they are allowed to go unchecked. These problems include:

(a) shortage of staff at the nurse/midwife level, with the work consequently being left to aides who are not adequately trained for it;

(b) lack of supervision, which may arise because of lack of transport to distant facilities, or because of pressure of work on the designated supervisor, or sometimes because he or she has not been properly trained to supervise;

---

[1] Smith, J. B. et al. *Hospital deaths in a high-risk obstetric population.* Unpublished Family Health International document, 1985.

(c) lack of essential equipment at clinics—not only of haemoglobinometers for detecting anaemia, but also of sphygmomanometers, weighing scales, and the means of testing urine, and of continuously available stocks of such items as ferrous sulfate tablets or tetanus toxoid;

(d) under-utilization by pregnant women of existing facilities.

Another major problem is the failure of the system to provide adequate prenatal care to cover the population (see Table 8.1). This has serious implications, since a disproportionate number of maternal deaths and serious injuries often occur among women arriving at hospital in emergency, with complications that could have been prevented.

Table 8.1. Proportion of pregnant women receiving prenatal care[a] and annual number of births, selected developing countries

| Region/Country | Coverage of prenatal care (%) | Total number of births (in millions) |
|---|---|---|
| AFRICA | | |
| Madagascar | 33 (1979) | 0.39 |
| Congo | 35 (1970) | 0.07 |
| Zimbabwe | 37 (1980) | 0.35 |
| Kenya | 63 (1979) | 0.88 |
| Botswana | 82 (1984) | 0.04 |
| Gambia | 90 (1978) | 0.03 |
| LATIN AMERICA | | |
| Honduras | 20 (1977) | 0.17 |
| Ecuador | 33 (1977) | 0.33 |
| Dominican Republic | 48 (1972) | 0.21 |
| Venezuela | 68 (1977) | 0.20 |
| Jamaica | 78 (1981) | 0.25 |
| Colombia | 81 (1977) | 0.81 |
| ASIA | | |
| Islamic Republic of Iran | 5 (1982) | 1.65 |
| Iraq | 35 (1979) | 0.60 |
| Thailand | 33 (1977) | 1.47 |
| Indonesia | 35 (1980) | 4.77 |
| India | 45 (1981) | 23.24 |
| Turkey | 50 (1979) | 1.55 |
| Republic of Korea | 76 (1980) | 0.95 |
| Malaysia | 80 (1980) | 0.45 |
| Philippines | 83 (1970) | 1.72 |
| China | 98 (1980) | 20.25 |

[a] At least one visit to a trained person.

Source: Coverage of maternity care. A tabulation of available information. Unpublished WHO document. FHE/85.1.

## Maternity waiting homes

Maternity waiting homes effectively bridge the gap between the prenatal period and the onset of labour. They are places close to hospitals where women from rural areas some distance away can stay for a while before the expected onset of labour. Frequently women are accompanied by members of their family. Maternity waiting homes are particularly useful for women who are thought to be at special risk and who can thereby avoid the dangers and difficulties of beginning what may be a long journey after labour has begun or some emergency has occurred. These waiting areas or homes need not be elaborate. In some cases communities have built their own; sometimes, as in Cuba for instance, large vacant houses have been taken over for this purpose, while elsewhere families living near a hospital have accommodated women from more distant locations (J. Rodriguez, unpublished information, 1986).

Such facilities are in use today in many parts of Africa and Latin America, as indeed they were at the turn of the century in France and Sweden and no doubt in other parts of Europe and North America, where people lived far from maternity services. Maternity waiting homes are far less expensive to run than hospitals, since in most places the women and any relatives accompanying them provide their own bedding and food, and look after themselves and each other.

This is the case at the "maternity village" attached to Ituk Mbang hospital near Uyo in eastern Nigeria (8), where women at risk can be accommodated during the last trimester of pregnancy. Here they are under medical supervision, they receive iron and vitamins and antimalarial drugs, and are taught about good nutrition and child care. Once labour starts or complications occur, the women can be transferred to the hospital for skilled care. The presence of the maternity village has been one of the factors responsible for bringing down the maternal mortality rate at Ituk Mbang hospital from 10 per 1000 deliveries, to less than 1 per 1000, and the stillbirth rate from 116 to 20 per 1000 deliveries.

In Cali, Colombia, the *casa hogar*, a purpose-built maternity waiting home, takes women from rural areas as well as from the extensive urban shanty town whose access to health services is made difficult not by distance but by economic and cultural constraints. Recognizing the difficulty most women have in taking time away from home and family, the health team and members of the local community between them help to arrange alternative family support.[1]

There have been few formal evaluations of the effect of maternity waiting homes on maternal mortality, but many anecdotal accounts similar to those cited above give a favourable impression of their value.

## Care during childbirth

A basic essential of maternal health care is that every woman should have the assistance of a trained person during labour, whether birth takes place at home or in hospital. However, this is very far from being the case (see Table 8.2). Around 1983, while practically all births in developed countries were attended by a qualified midwife or doctor, only 64% of births in Latin America, 49% in Asia (even taking into account the 98% in China), and only 34% in Africa were attended by trained persons. There is obviously a long way to go in the training and deployment of more midwives before even the modest objective of giving every woman in labour the chance of skilled attendance can be achieved. In such circumstances the upgrading of the existing traditional birth attendants (TBAs) and their incorporation into the national health system has been considered by many as the most practical response to the problem. After all, industrialized countries took this course of action at the turn of the century, as did China after 1950.

### The traditional birth attendant and the health service

In most societies cultural and spiritual aspects of pregnancy and childbirth have a strong influence on behaviour. It is important that health care providers are aware of these aspects so that they can organize services that are appropriate and acceptable to the people. Unfortunately, there are usually limited opportunities for health personnel to explore the sociocultural context of childbirth.

One of the most important arguments in favour of greater collaboration between the traditional birth attendant (TBA) and the health services is that it is a way of bridging the

---

[1] Rodriguez, J. *Summary of the maternity home (casa hogar) project.* Unpublished document, 1986.

Table 8.2. Percentage of births attended by trained personnel, by region, around 1983

| Region | No. of births (millions) | Percentage attended by trained personnel |
|---|---|---|
| *Developing countries* | | |
| Africa | 23.4 | 34 |
|   Northern Africa | 4.8 | 31 |
|   Eastern Africa | 7.0 | 29 |
|   Central Africa | 2.6 | 29 |
|   Western Africa | 7.6 | 36 |
|   Southern Africa | 1.4 | 65 |
| Asia | 73.9 | 49 |
|   Southern Asia | 35.6 | 20 |
|   Western Asia | 4.1 | 61 |
|   Southeastern Asia | 12.4 | 53 |
|   East Asia | 21.8 | 93 |
| Latin America | 12.6 | 64 |
|   Central America | 3.7 | 51 |
|   Caribbean | 0.9 | 58 |
|   Tropical South America | 7.1 | 69 |
|   Temperate South America | 0.9 | 89 |
| Oceania | 0.2 | 34 |
| Total (developing countries) | 110.1 | 48 |
| *Developed countries* | | |
| North America | 4.4 | 100 |
| Europe | 6.9 | 97 |
|   Northern Europe | 1.0 | 100 |
|   Western Europe | 1.8 | 100 |
|   Eastern Europe | 1.9 | 99 |
|   Southern Europe | 2.2 | 93 |
| USSR | 5.1 | _[a] |
| *Total (developed countries)* | *18.2[b]* | *98[c]* |
| *World total* | *128.3* | *55* |

[a] *Data for the USSR are not available.*
[b] *Includes Australia, Japan, and New Zealand.*
[c] *This figure is calculated on the assumption that the figure for the USSR is the same as that for Eastern Europe.*

gap between what are often two very different cultures. Much has been published on this topic (*9, 10, 11*) and in the last 15–20 years a great deal of collaborative effort between national governments and WHO, UNFPA and UNICEF has gone into the training of TBAs so that they can be incorporated in the health care system. Results have been mixed: while there have been successes, there have also been disappointments, and certain lessons have been learnt.

1. The most commonly cited reason for unsatisfactory results from TBA training is lack of supervision after training. This is frequently because provision for supervision is not built into the training programme from the start. Inadequate resources are allocated to it, and sometimes it is a duty expected of someone whose time is already fully committed. Without supervision, TBAs easily become disillusioned with their new role and may revert to their old practices.

2. Follow-up of TBAs immediately after training also appears crucial in motivating them to put their new knowledge into practice. This is when TBAs are making the adjustment from their former role to their new one, and they particularly need support at this time.

3. The issues of a stipend during training and subsequent reward for the services of the TBA need careful consideration. Such payments should take account of the extra responsibility that the TBA is expected to carry and should be culturally acceptable both to her and to the community that she serves. In some programmes TBAs are provided with a maternity kit free of charge as part of their reward. A TBA training programme in Andhra Pradesh (*12*) found little enthusiasm amongst TBAs initially when they received a stipend of 3 rupees (Rs) per day over the training period, and no maternity kit. As part of the subsequent reassessment of the programme the stipend was raised to Rs 300 per month; TBAs were provided with a maternity kit, and they were entitled to a payment of Rs 2 for every delivery conducted, provided that it was registered with the health services. In the Sierra Leone programme, 75% of TBAs questioned said they had encountered problems over the issue of payment.

4. Dissatisfaction with arrangements for replenishing maternity kits is another common problem. Adequate provision should therefore be made for replenishment, or trainers should discuss possible substitutes for items in the kits that would be readily available locally.

5. The length and content of training needs careful consideration. Most TBAs have limited time to spend on this activity. It is important that trainers discover from TBAs the knowledge and beliefs that have been the basis of their traditional practice, and adapt the training accor-

dingly. Many TBAs are illiterate, so training should be as practical and participatory as possible.

6. Experience shows that respect for the TBA from the health professionals is very important to success because there is a good deal of contact between the trained TBA and the health service. In the Sierra Leone programme TBAs had a reasonably good relationship with medical field staff, but a poor relationship with hospital staff, and this was considered a regrettable constraint. Issues of professional sensibility therefore need to be understood and treated with tact and respect.

7. Care should be taken to ensure that efforts to train TBAs never take precedence over, or are undertaken at the expense of, endeavours to supply more adequate midwifery and obstetric care to people in obvious need of these services.

By the early 1980s around 82% of countries had training programmes for TBAs compared with 37% a decade earlier. An example of a successful programme is provided by a scheme in north-east Brazil (3). Believing on the one hand that fundamental change could not be hurried, and on the other that there was too much interference with childbirth in modern obstetric practice in Brazil, the late professor of obstetrics at Fortaleza hospital, Dr Galba Araujo, set out to improve the quality of care given by the TBAs and to provide support from the health service only where necessary. Making use of health buildings abandoned through lack of funds, staff or commitment, he created in the early 1970s a series of satellite maternity units centred on Fortaleza hospital. Dr Araujo gave basic training to the TBAs and got the natural leaders among them to organize 24-hour coverage at the units for local women in labour. Arrangements were made for the units to be visited by professional nurses several times a week, and obstetricians from the hospital visited generally at weekends. Any TBA who wished to use the unit to deliver one of her patients could do so. The TBAs were paid by the health service, and funds were set aside to pay for transport to the hospital for any woman needing professional care.

Respect for tradition was one of the key elements in the programme. Professional staff would not interfere in the process of delivery unless problems beyond the scope of the TBA arose. The TBAs were taught to put up an intravenous drip, but otherwise reliance on modern drugs and technology was avoided. The programme showed good results from the beginning: there were no maternal deaths among the first 500 deliveries at the satellite maternity units.

## Appropriate technology for TBAs

The minimum requirements for the conduct of a safe delivery are:

(*a*) a clean surface on which delivery can take place;

(*b*) clean hands of the birth attendant;

(*c*) clean cutting of the umbilical cord;

(*d*) keeping the baby warm immediately after delivery.

The teaching of simple hygiene principles—known as the "three cleans"—to TBAs in China in the 1950s did much to reduce the number of deaths from puerperal sepsis (and also neonatal tetanus); this should be the basis of TBA training generally.

Hygienic practices can be encouraged by the provision of maternity kits as mentioned earlier, and there is no reason why such kits should not be made widely available—to anyone attending a birth or to mothers themselves, perhaps through local stores.

The minimum contents of a maternity kit are:[1]

(*a*) soap;

(*b*) sticks for cleaning under the nails of the attendant;

(*c*) string or cotton tapes for tying the umbilical cord; these should be washed, boiled and preferably sun-dried to ensure sterility (3 or 4 tapes at least, and extras in case one is dropped or otherwise contaminated);

(*d*) a cord-cutting instrument—a razor blade (broken in half to discourage anyone from using it for other purposes) or

---

[1] *A simplified childbirth kit for primary health care. Report of a working group meeting, Sri Lanka, November 1985.* Unpublished WHO document FHE/86.4.

split bamboo (boiled and dried before use); rusty blades should **never** be used;

(*e*) cottonwool balls;

(*f*) plastic sheeting or a new woven mat to provide a clean surface for delivery;

(*g*) two pieces of clean cloth: one for wiping the baby and one for wiping the mother's perineum after delivery; these cloths should be washed and sun-dried between deliveries.

It is an advantage if items in the kit can be made or supplied locally because this lessens the dependence of the TBA on her supervisors for replenishing her equipment.

There are certain other procedures whose more widespread use even at the periphery would help to control some of the major causes of maternal mortality.[1] One of these is the use of the partograph, on which a record is kept of the progress of labour.[2] By providing a visual record of the progress, this helps the attendant to detect possible problems, particularly cephalopelvic disproportion, early on.

This is not suitable for use by the TBA, even in simplified form, because it requires manual examination of the mother, but midwives at all levels can be taught to use it effectively. It is generally considered to be an invaluable aid to all who attend deliveries.

The main features recorded on the partograph are:

(*a*) the condition of the fetus: heart rate, condition of the liquor, degree of moulding of the head;

(*b*) the progress of labour: rate of cervical dilatation, rate of descent of presenting part, frequency and duration of uterine contractions;

(*c*) the condition of the mother: blood pressure, pulse and temperature, condition of urine, any therapy given, etc.

---

[1] *Prevention of maternal mortality. Report of a WHO interregional meeting, Geneva, 11–15 November 1985.* Unpublished WHO document FHE/86.1.

[2] *The partograph: a managerial tool for the prevention of prolonged labour.* Unpublished WHO documents, WHO/MCH/88.3 and WHO/MCH/88.4.

## Access to life-saving obstetric care

Studies of maternal mortality and morbidity in the Third World frequently identify lack of access to life-saving treatment in emergencies as the single most critical failing in the maternal health system. Though it has been repeatedly stressed in this book that the complication immediately preceding a maternal death is by no means the whole cause, there is no doubt that this last line of defence is present and functioning in countries where maternal mortality is low, and is absent, inaccessible or malfunctioning in countries where maternal mortality is high. It is mainly the difference in access to well staffed and equipped hospitals that accounts for the often marked differences in maternal mortality rates between urban and rural areas of the same country. This pattern can be seen even in a rapidly industrializing country like China where much progress has been made in maternal health care (13). Here a maternal mortality rate of 59 per 100 000 live births has been recorded for rural areas compared with 25 in urban areas of 21 provinces.

The more equitable provision of care for obstetric emergencies is a part of the system that has long been neglected, perhaps because of the many difficulties involved. For instance, it is known that few doctors are willing to serve in isolated rural areas. In some countries in Africa, for example, 50–75% of physicians are located in the capital city, where only about 10% of the people live. Furthermore, it is believed that the building of new hospitals would represent an impossible financial burden to governments. So indeed it might be if this were the only solution, but it is not. Much can be done to improve access to existing services, and some means of achieving this have already been discussed. For example, the patient living in the countryside can reach life-saving care "soon enough" by beginning the journey earlier (prompted by the partograph), or before the emergency happens (the maternity waiting home), or by beginning her journey in a better general state of health (following prevention of severe anaemia, control of pre-eclampsia, antibiotic cover, etc.).

Even so, emergencies happen, and many are neither predictable nor preventable. There is a great need, therefore, to address the problem of transportation; this can often be done through a combination of local government action and mobilization of the community itself. One possibility is for certain villages to have access to a telephone or police radio communication in an emergency to summon a vehicle from the district administrative centre. If, as is often the case, no health department vehicle is available, it should be possible to requisition any government vehicle.

A maternal health scheme in southern Ethiopia, for example, makes use of messengers who will run and walk for up to three hours from a village on request of the TBA who is part of the primary health care team.[1] When the messenger has alerted the sisters at the primary health care post that there is a woman in difficulties, they leave for the village—or as near as they can get to it—in a motor vehicle to transfer the woman to the first referral level of the health service.

There are many other possibilities, such as having recognized points along a road where commercial vehicles can be flagged down. There are few places in the world, no matter how poor, where there is not some possibility of improving the provision of emergency transport. It is the people who are affected who are most likely to devise an effective solution to the problem, but they will often need the support and cooperation of local government.

Another possible answer is an obstetric flying squad. This is particularly suited to urban and periurban areas where there are both roads and good telephone communications. However, in 1975 a description was given of a modified version of the flying squad in use in a rural area of Nigeria where communications were poor and the service relied on a messenger being sent from the village to the state maternity hospital at Katsina to call for help. On receiving a call, one or more members of the nursing staff would set out in an ambulance for the village, taking with them a prepared set of equipment in a box. The box was specially designed to be light enough to be carried by one person—an important consideration, since many people lived beyond the reach of the ambulance, and the staff had to walk the extra distance before a "rickshaw ambulance" was designed to improve the system. Emergency equipment included oxygen, an intravenous drip, fresh water, soap, sterile dressings and a selection of obstetric instruments. Staff were given a year's training in the emergency management of the three principal causes of death in the area: obstructed labour, haemorrhage, and eclampsia. At the home of the patient they would

---

[1] WHO/IBRD/UNFPA. Safe Motherhood Conference press kit, 1987.

prepare her for the journey to hospital in the ambulance, and collect blood donors to accompany her (*14*).

Improving access to existing hospitals by whatever means is undoubtedly part of the solution. However, after careful consideration of reports from some twenty countries, a WHO meeting on the prevention of maternal mortality, seeing that most deaths occurred in the rural areas of developing countries, concluded that a major part of the solution lay in extending to the periphery the network of places where the essential life-saving obstetric functions could be undertaken. It adopted the axioms that **health services should be made available as close to people's homes as possible**, and that **any health care procedure should be carried out by the least trained person who is competent to perform it safely and well**.[1]

Very often what is needed to provide essential services is not a new hospital but the upgrading of an existing rural or district hospital or health centre which already has maternity beds for normal deliveries but is unable to deal with grave emergencies. Hand in hand with the upgrading of facilities goes a reassessment of the role and capabilities of health personnel.

A WHO working group subsequently defined the essential obstetric functions at first referral level[2] necessary to save maternal lives, and specified the main requirements for carrying out these functions in terms of staff, training and supervision, physical facilities, equipment and supplies (*24*). The essential obstetric functions were defined as:

1. *Surgical functions*: caesarean section; surgical treatment of sepsis; repairs of high vaginal and cervical tears and uterine rupture; removal of ectopic pregnancy; evacuation of uterus in incomplete abortion.

2. *Anaesthetic functions*.

3. *Medical treatment*: treatment of shock; intravenous administration of iron in severe anaemia or blood loss;

---

[1] *Prevention of maternal mortality. Report of a WHO interregional meeting, Geneva, 11–15 November 1985.* Unpublished WHO document FHE/86.1.
[2] The first referral level means the district or subdistrict hospital or health centre to which a woman identified prenatally as definitely high-risk is referred, or to which a woman is usually sent when she is in serious difficulty or in an emergency in pregnancy, childbirth or immediately after.

control of sepsis; control of hypertensive disorders of pregnancy and eclamptic fits.

4. *Blood replacement.*

5. *Manual and/or assessment functions*: manual removal of placenta; vacuum extraction to hasten delivery in second stage of labour; use of partograph.

6. *Family planning support*: tubal ligation and vasectomy, fitting of intrauterine devices.

7. *Management of women at high risk*, through maternity villages or homes.

8. *Neonatal special care*, including resuscitation, thermal control and feeding. (Though clearly not for the purpose of reducing maternal mortality, it is difficult to imagine a facility which provides maternal health care without provision of some special care for the newborn. This must therefore be included for practical planning purposes.)

## Health manpower

Expanding the provision of maternity health care means making the most of existing resources in personnel just as much as in facilities. The guiding principle "any health care procedure should be carried out by the least trained person who is competent to perform it safely and well" requires a fundamental reassessment of the present duties and potential capabilities of personnel, mainly at the lower levels of the health service, where workers are more numerous and most accessible to the women who need them.

However, because it means questioning the often long-standing traditions that have reserved certain procedures for those at higher levels of the service, it can be an extremely difficult process. It requires careful planning, changes in basic training (and cooperation and retraining of personnel already in the field) and new job descriptions. (The need for the latter is often overlooked, leaving people without a clear definition of their responsibilities and limits, and thereby undermining self-confidence and initiative.)

Already there is much variety between countries as to who carries out which functions. For example, caesarean section, which is the exclusive preserve of obstetricians in some countries, is performed by specially trained medical assistants in others. This is the case in Malawi and in parts of Zaire where nurse-practitioners can undergo training in obstetric surgery and subsequently perform caesarean section (15).

Decisions on who should do what should take account of the level of demand (or need) for a particular life-saving intervention, and the chances a patient has of receiving care under the existing system. The consequences of inflexibility may be many unnecessary deaths.

As mentioned earlier, highly trained personnel are often reluctant to work in rural areas. This situation may be exacerbated by the fact that training is predominantly urban-based, urban-oriented and frequently western-influenced. The problem that this reluctance causes as regards extending services to isolated communities can be overcome to some extent by recognizing the value of middle-level workers—particularly, in this case, enrolled midwives—who usually train in peripheral areas and do not aspire to a job in the city. However, in some countries the search for greater professionalism has led to a raising of the educational requirements for entry into training, and a phasing-out of this level of midwife (16). Whether or not this is a desirable trend needs to be reassessed in the light of results: does it afford better care for the rural population, or open a new gap in provision?

As has been emphasized before, the concept of the health team is very important: personnel, from the obstetrician or physician at first referral level to the health worker or TBA at the front line, should work in cooperation, with support and supervision being offered all down the line. For this to be possible, the barriers that separate categories of personnel—often erected during initial training—need to come down. There are several ways of achieving this. For example, teamwork could become part of the training curriculum of different health workers, or students from different courses could be brought together for practical fieldwork as a team.

Crucial to the success of teamwork is good supervision. Health personnel at the periphery need regular encourage-ment, technical guidance and instruction. Besides, good morale throughout a team helps to ensure that all members are fulfilling their potential and not referring cases unneces-sarily. As J. V. Larsen, Professor of Obstetrics at Eshowe Hospital, Zululand, says (17):

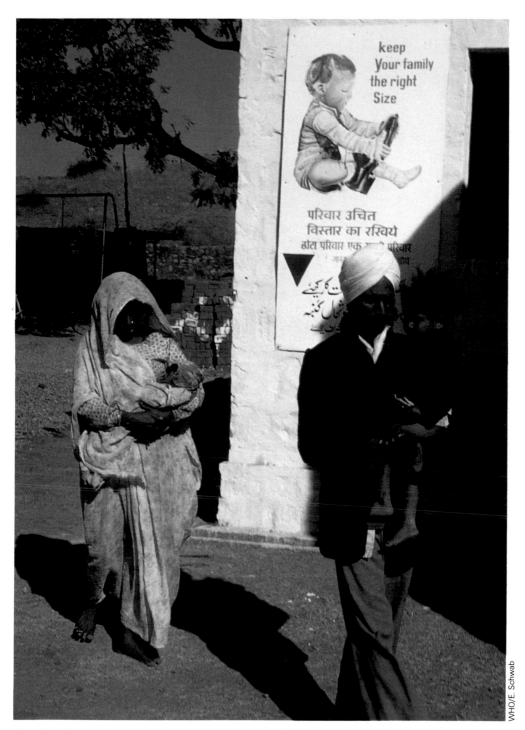

On the poster:

keep
Your family
the right
Size

परिवार उचित
विस्तार का रखिये
छोटा परिवार एक ... परिवार

WHO/E. Schwab

**Family planning services can contribute to reducing maternal mortality by helping to create healthy conditions for childbearing.**

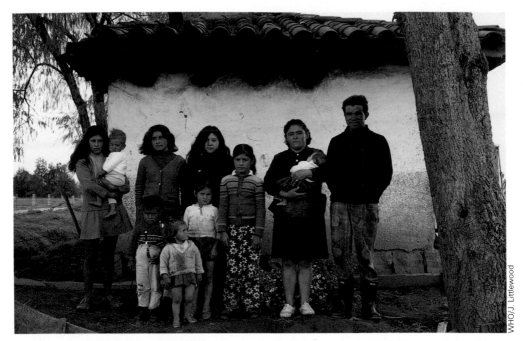

In some societies, bearing children is one of the few ways available to a woman of enhancing her social status and gaining prestige.

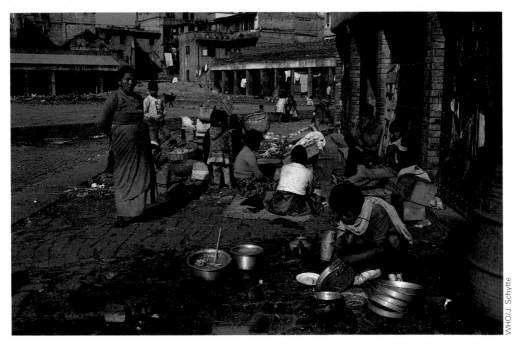

Each year, millions of women with unwanted pregnancies resort to the services of back-street abortionists, at enormous risk to their health.

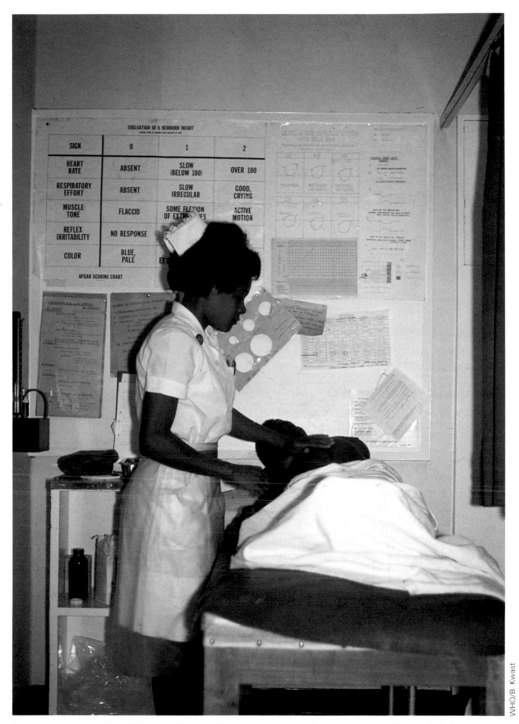

**Every woman should have the assistance of a trained person during labour.**

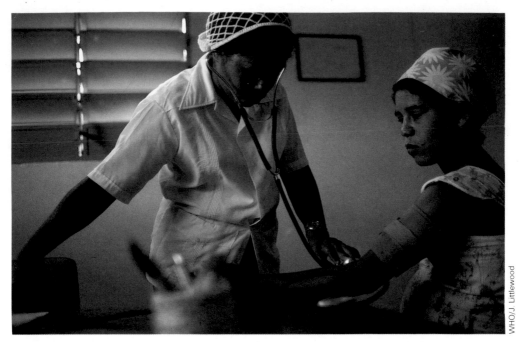

**Basic prenatal care permits early detection and treatment of conditions that could otherwise prove life-threatening.**

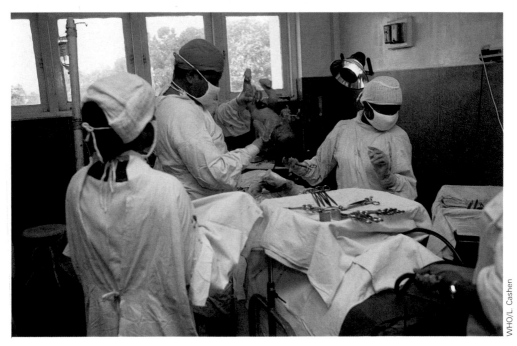

**A happy outcome to pregnancy and childbirth may depend on prompt and effective intervention by health service personnel.**

Clearly it is wasteful and frustrating for a doctor who sets out to provide a high standard of care [in a developing country] to confine his activities to the well-equipped hospital. No amount of technology or Herculean effort expended there compensates for a poor quality of care at lower and wider levels of the triangle. The doctor must involve himself in the supervision of every peripheral unit that refers to the base hospital if he is to be successful in providing the highest quality of care possible with the facilities available to him.

Like health education, supervision requires commitment from the top; it will not happen unless provision is made for it in time and resources. Furthermore, it should not be delegated to someone who is not familiar with an area, the communities being served and the strengths and weaknesses of the health care providers. The relationship between supervisor and supervised should be one of mutual respect and confidence, so that problems can be discussed, not covered up, and staff remain willing to learn from their more experienced colleagues.

It is also important that a supervisor has respect for the chain of authority and does not bypass one level to talk directly to personnel at another if this is likely to cause ill-will.

## Postnatal care

There are several important aspects of postnatal care, one of which may be life-saving. This is the early treatment of puerperal sepsis. Antibiotic treatment alone is sufficient in over 80% of cases if instituted within four days of the onset of fever,[1] though increasing microbial resistance to antibiotics does pose a problem. Those who attend women postnatally must know the signs of puerperal sepsis (fever, lower abdominal pain or tenderness, excessive or offensive lochia). Treatment should not be delayed, otherwise surgery may be needed later to drain pus or, as too often happens, the patient may develop generalized septicaemia and die. If a pelvic abscess is suspected, early drainage of pus is advisable before generalized peritonitis occurs. Moreover, blood transfusion will be necessary if sepsis has caused a serious fall in the haemoglobin level.

---

[1] Winikoff, B. *Medical services to save mothers' lives. Feasible approaches to reducing maternal mortality.* Paper presented at the Safe Motherhood Conference, Nairobi, 10–13 February 1987.

Another important aspect is encouragement, and help where needed, with breast-feeding. Advice should be given on a proper diet for the mother and the need for rest especially where traditional customs are in conflict with the health needs of mother or child. For example, in parts of India, colostrum is widely thought to be poisonous, and breast milk is therefore discarded for the first two or three days postpartum (*16*). In Sokoto State, Nigeria, the TBA tests breast milk by observing its reaction on hot metal. If it coagulates it is considered unsuitable, and other methods of feeding the baby are suggested (*18*).

A third important aspect of postnatal care is often missing. This consists of discussion with the mother concerning the length of time she would like to elapse before she has another child. The discussion should include an explanation by the health worker of how an interval of at least two years would benefit the woman herself, the newborn infant and the next child. If the mother wishes to use contraception, the health worker should advise her on a method that does not interfere with breast-feeding, and help her to obtain the necessary supplies.

## Under-utilization of services

As has been frequently mentioned in this book, the existence of facilities for maternal health care does not necessarily mean that they will be used—even by women who have been expressly advised to use them (see also Chapter 4). In some cases the explanation is simple and obvious: the clinic or hospital is too far from a woman's home and she lacks the time, transport, or possibly the money to reach it.

Alternatively, she may not appreciate the service it offers. According to a study in Zimbabwe, for instance, women in a particular rural area were prepared to accept prenatal care from the formal health services but preferred to deliver their child at home (*19*). The people made a clear distinction between physical health and hygiene, which they saw as the domain of the formal system, and spiritual and moral health, which were the domain of the informal health system. In the case of childbirth, the spiritual and moral needs of the newborn were given the highest priority by the villagers, who were reluctant therefore to deliver in hospital.

A recent study of women's perceptions determining the use of MCH services in Bangladesh identified the following typical reasons for non-use (20):

— MCH centres are seen as places to which one goes only if one has problems;

— home is the best place for delivery;

— delivery at the MCH centre is a matter of shame and the clinic environment is not congenial;

— healthy women and healthy babies need not be taken to centres or doctors;

— long distance and lack of company for visiting the clinic;

— long waiting time for services;

— inadequate supply or inferior quality of medicines;

— unconcerned attitude and rude behaviour of clinic personnel;

— demand for money for services;

— unfavourable attitude of husbands/relatives to delivery at the health centre.

A report on maternal death in the southern highlands of the United Republic of Tanzania stated that women tended not to visit the prenatal clinic until fairly late in pregnancy because they were motivated to seek attention mainly by a visible swelling of the abdomen. For a woman to attend such a clinic simply because she had not had a period for several months was almost unknown (21).

There is, moreover, a general tendency for women who are unhappy about being pregnant to neglect their special health needs, perhaps because they are reluctant to admit the reality of their situation to either themselves or others. Research in Ethiopia, for instance, revealed that only a small number of women with unwanted pregnancy sought prenatal care and most delivered either at home or in an MCH clinic where services were free (5).

The implications of these few examples are clear: those responsible for planning maternal health services must take full account of a wide variety of influences on women's decision-making if the services are going to be effective. This will also mean designing facilities that are culturally acceptable, such as maternity wards that respect the intense need for privacy in Muslim communities, or the desire to have family and friends around if that is the custom (8).

## The need for a linked system

At the Safe Motherhood Conference held in Nairobi in February 1987, it was stated that: "No maternal health programme can work effectively through action at one level only. Even if all women could deliver in well staffed and equipped hospitals, some way would be needed to identify and transport them to hospital in time. And no matter how effective community-based care for pregnant women might be, there will always be some irreducible minimum number of women who are likely to die if not delivered or treated in hospital" (22).

This is indeed true, and there are disappointments ahead for health planners who stake all on one single course of action—on family planning, or on training TBAs, or on primary health care—at the expense of others. If it is to succeed in a speedy and substantial reduction in maternal mortality and morbidity, maternal health care (including family planning) needs to be a linked system, operating at different levels and at different points in the reproductive cycle.

The adaptation, selection and balance of different interventions depend on the particular circumstances of each country, such as its fertility patterns, the extent, distribution and causes of maternal mortality and the degree to which existing health services meet or could meet the needs, as well as on financial, social and physical considerations. There is an acute need in many countries for an assessment of unmet needs in maternal health care, and for finding ways of meeting them, as far as possible with existing resources.

In order to do this it is necessary first to identify deficiencies in the system as it stands. This can be accomplished relatively simply by a review committee using existing data on the health needs of the people (including special risk groups and risk factors) and the coverage and use of services, and augmenting this information with a brief survey at household level of the performance of the services.

Sometimes the problems that become apparent from analysis of information can be resolved quickly and with only minor changes in the existing system. Alternatively expertise from outside and perhaps new resources may be required for a . solution.

However it is handled, evaluation and problem-solving should be a "bottom up" process, starting with the consumers and providers at the periphery, and not a "top down" one that starts with a high-level workshop.

An example of this method of problem-solving is furnished by Malaysia.[1] In Kedah State, poor management of high-risk pregnancies was identified by a health team from the district as a particular problem. The district team was taking part in an experiment organized by the Director-General of Health Services in Malaysia to find ways of assessing and solving problems at the level at which they occur, rather than automatically appealing to the Ministry for help. The team was given expert guidance during a 9-day workshop, conducted by the Institute of Public Health, on gathering data, analysing the problem and designing a solution, which they then had to implement and finally to evaluate over a period of 9 months.

As a result, better records of high-risk pregnancies were kept, marked with a blue tag for easy reference and regular follow-up. Efforts were intensified to ensure that professional attendants, rather than TBAs, were present at the birth and an obstetric flying squad was set up. In addition, family members were advised of the indications of high risk and the need under such circumstances for professional care during delivery. These changes in management of high-risk pregnancies quickly yielded results: during the seven months of 1986 under review there were no deaths in the district due to postpartum haemorrhage, whereas in 1985 there were seven such deaths.

## Conclusion

It has been estimated that the incidence of complications of pregnancy in developing countries may be as high as 30%.

---

[1] Sapirie, S. A. *Action health systems research through district health team problem solving. The Malaysian experience.* Presentation to the Workshop and Seminar on Methods and Experience in Planning for Health, Gothenburg, Sweden, 1–12 June 1987.

Much can be done to reduce the proportion by ensuring that women arrive at pregnancy in a healthy condition as a result of adequate nutrition and attention to their health needs from childhood onwards. But such preventive measures will never be enough to prevent maternal death, as a rare example shows. A study between 1975 and 1982 of a religious group in the USA who accepted no medical intervention whatsoever during pregnancy and childbirth, recorded a maternal mortality rate of 870 per 100 000 live births, though the women were well nourished and in good health generally (23). This rate was almost 100 times higher than that for the rest of the population in the state in which the religious group lived, whose health status was comparable but who accepted maternal health care.

The provision of good quality maternal health services is essential to save lives. It is true, too, that funds for health care are most limited where the needs are greatest. But this is no reason to turn away from the challenge. Experience has shown that much can be done to expand provision of care at very little extra cost by making better use of facilities and personnel already available. For this approach, fresh awareness, the willingness to break with traditional patterns of thought and action, and above all commitment are needed.

# References

1. MAHLER, H. The safe motherhood initiative: a call to action. *Lancet*, 1(8534): 668–670 (1987).
2. SCHMIDT, H. J. & KERR, D. Motivation for primary health care in Machinga district. *Medical quarterly (Malawi)*, 4(1): 17–21 (1987).
3. POTTS, M. Childbirth in Fortaleza. *Profiles (Kellog Foundation)*, 4(2): 11–14 (1981).
4. GREENWOOD, A. ET AL. A prospective study of pregnancy in a rural area of the Gambia, West Africa. *Bulletin of the World Health Organization*, 65(5): 635–644 (1987).
5. KWAST, B. E. ET AL. *Report on maternal health in Addis Ababa*. Addis Ababa, Swedish Save the Children Federation, 1984.
6. ADRIASOLA, E. ET AL. Influencia del control prenatal sobre la morbimortalidad materna y perinatal. *Boletín de la Oficina Sanitaria Panamericana*, 83(5): 413–424 (1977).
7. HARRISON, K. A. Childbearing, health and social priorities. A survey of 22,774 consecutive births in Zaria, Northern Nigeria. *British journal of obstetrics and gynaecology*, Supplement No. 5 (1985).

8. STEWART D. B. & LAWSON, J. B. The organization of obstetric services. In: *Obstetrics and gynaecology in the tropics and developing countries*. London, Edward Arnold, 1967, pp. 305–313.

9. MANGAY-MAGLACAS, A. & PIZURKI, H. *The traditional birth attendant in seven countries: case studies in utilization and training.* Geneva, World Health Organization, 1981 (Public Health Papers, No. 75).

10. WORLD HEALTH ORGANIZATION. *Traditional birth attendants: a field guide to their training, evaluation and articulation with health services.* Geneva, 1979 (WHO Offset Publication, No. 44).

11. LEEDHAM, E. Traditional birth attendants. *International journal of gynaecology and obstetrics*, **23**: 249–274 (1985).

12. MANGAY-MAGLACAS, A. & SIMONS, J., ed. *The potential of the traditional birth attendant.* Geneva, World Health Organization, 1986 (WHO Offset Publication No. 95).

13. ZHANG, L. & DING, H. China: Analysis of cause and rate of regional maternal deaths in 21 provinces, municipalities and autonomous regions. *Chinese journal of obstetrics and gynaecology*, **21**(4): 195–197 (1986).

14. ST GEORGE, I. The obstetric flying squad: a method of reducing maternal mortality and morbidity in developing countries. *Tropical doctor*, **5**: 410–415 (1975).

15. WHITE, S. M. ET AL. Emergency obstetric surgery performed by nurses in Zaire. *Lancet*, **2**(8559): 612–613 (1987).

16. PHILPOTT, R. H., ed. *Maternity services in the developing world— what the community needs.* London, Royal College of Obstetricians and Gynaecologists, 1980.

17. LARSEN, J. V. Supervision of peripheral obstetric units. *Tropical doctor*, **17**: 77–81 (1987).

18. ITYAVYAR, D. A. A traditional midwife practice, Sokoto State, Nigeria. *Social science and medicine*, **18**(6): 497–501 (1984).

19. MUTAMBIRWA, J. Pregnancy, childbirth, mother and child care among the indigenous people of Zimbabwe. *International journal of gynaecology and obstetrics*, **23**(4): 275–285 (1985).

20. RAHMAN, S. *Determinants of the utilization of maternal and child health services.* Dhaka, National Institute of Population Research and Training and USAID, 1981.

21. PRICE, T. G. Preliminary report on maternal deaths in the southern highlands of Tanzania in 1983. *Journal of obstetrics and gynaecology of Eastern and Central Africa*, **3**: 103–110 (1984).

22. HERZ, B. & MEASHAM, A. R. *The safe motherhood initiative: proposals for action.* Washington, DC, World Bank, 1987.

23. KAUNITZ, A. M. ET AL. Perinatal and maternal mortality in a religious group avoiding obstetric care. *American journal of obstetrics and gynecology*, **150**(7): 826–831 (1984).

24. *Essential elements of obstetric care at first referral level.* Geneva, World Health Organization, in press.

# Chapter 9

# THE ROLE OF FAMILY PLANNING IN PREVENTING MATERNAL DEATHS

---

> Like pure water and like nutritious food, family planning is
> essential for good health (*1*).

Somewhere in Africa an unmarried teenager becomes
pregnant. Forced to drop out of school early, she faces an
uncertain future. In Latin America a pregnant woman in her
late thirties sits outside her hut watching the four surviving
children of the ten she has borne, playing in the afternoon
sun. In a small room many thousands of miles away in Asia,
another woman, faced with an unwanted pregnancy, has
decided she cannot go through with it, and is submitting to
the hazards of a backstreet abortion.

However diverse their circumstances and locations, these
women have something in common: an inability to control
their own fertility, and consequently a high degree of risk
that they will, sooner or later, suffer ill health or even death
as a result of pregnancy.

Because so many maternal deaths are a consequence of
unregulated fertility, family planning has a strong role to
play in saving lives. But, as things stand at present, family
planning is achieving only a fraction of its potential.
According to the World Fertility Survey (WFS) some 300
million couples who say they want no more children are not
practising contraception (*2*).

The lack of services and supplies is only part of the problem.
Because it touches upon the most private, personal and
poorly understood aspects of people's lives, family planning
needs to be very sensitive to local conditions if it is to be
effective. Unless it takes into account the attitude of a
particular community towards children and fertility, and the
patterns of decision-making as well as the customs and
beliefs surrounding sexual matters, much of the effort of any
programme will be wasted.

This chapter will look at family planning first from the point of view of what it might hypothetically achieve in terms of numbers of maternal lives saved. It will then focus on the practical issues of family planning: the present coverage and the unmet need; the design and delivery of services; and the attitudes and practices of those who are, or could be, their customers. And because the health of infants is so closely tied to that of mothers, this chapter will also touch upon the effects of family planning on child survival.

## The potential for saving lives

The number of maternal deaths in developing countries reflects two factors:

(*a*) a high risk for the individual woman in becoming pregnant and giving birth; and

(*b*) high fertility (i.e., the frequency with which women become pregnant).

Family planning has the potential to save lives on both counts, by enabling women to plan their pregnancies in such a way that they avoid becoming pregnant at an age or achieving a parity that carries additional risks, and by lowering fertility generally, i.e., by reducing the absolute number of pregnancies in the population. In addition, family planning can reduce the number of unwanted pregnancies and hence the number of illicit abortions and the deaths that these cause.

### Avoiding high-risk pregnancy

As has been shown in previous chapters, the safest period for a woman to bear children is between the ages of 20 and 35 years. The risk of death is significantly increased for women who become pregnant while still in their teens or after the age of 35. These differentials exist everywhere (see Fig 9.1), but the dangers are greatest where women are in poor general health and beyond the reach of good quality obstetric care. Under such circumstances the differentials compound an already high risk of dying from maternal causes.

A study in Bangladesh, for instance, found maternal mortality rates of 860 and 810 per 100 000 births for women of less than 19 years and women of 40–44 years respectively, compared with a rate of 380 per 100 000 for women aged

Fig. 9.1.  Maternal mortality by age, in the USA and Bangladesh

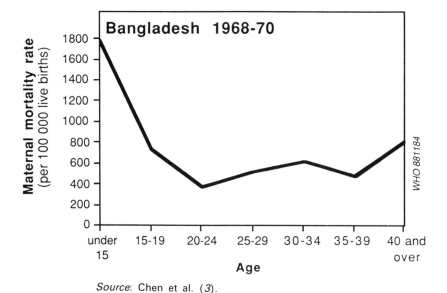

Source: Nortman (5).

Source: Chen et al. (3).

20–24 years (3). A maternal mortality rate of 474 per 100 000 births was recorded in Thailand in 1971 among women over 40, compared with a rate of 154 per 100 000 among women in their 20s (4). Even in the USA the rate for women aged 40–44 years was more than eight times higher than that for women in their early 20s (5).

In the world as a whole, more than one-third of all births are to mothers in their teens or over the age of 35 years (5), and between 12 and 18 million babies a year are born to teenagers (1,6). But these figures mask considerable variations between regions.

In addition to the age-related risk, there is an increased risk of maternal death associated with high parity. The second and third births are generally the safest for the mother; the mortality rate usually begins to rise with the fourth, and rises dramatically with the birth of the fifth and each subsequent child. Figures from Jamaica, for instance, showed that the risk of death for women having their fifth or subsequent delivery was about double that of women having their second, while for women having a tenth or higher-order birth the risk was almost threefold (7).

A birth interval of at least two years is generally recommended to allow a woman's body time to recover from the extra demands of pregnancy and lactation. Intervals shorter than this take a particularly heavy toll on women who are habitually overworked, undernourished and in poor health. The term "maternal depletion syndrome" has been used to describe their condition, but while it would seem likely that a relationship that affects maternal health should also affect maternal mortality, until now very little research has been done on the relationship of close birth intervals and the risk of maternal death. An analysis of all maternal deaths occurring in three hospitals in Bangkok in 1973 to 1977 showed that women with a previous birth interval of less than two years had a two-and-a-half times greater risk of dying than women with a longer birth interval.[1]

In summary, women run the least risk of pregnancy-related death and illness if they:

(*a*) refrain from starting their families until they have reached the age of at least 20;

(*b*) have no more than four children;

(*c*) have birth intervals of at least two years;

(*d*) do not have children after the age of 35 years.

---

[1] Rattanaporn, P. *The internal factors affecting maternal mortality.* Thesis, Mahidol University, Bangkok, 1980.

Encouraging women to observe such a pattern will have unquestionable benefits at the personal level, but this may not translate into a significant reduction in overall maternal mortality because, generally speaking, the large majority of births (and therefore deaths) occur outside these high-risk categories. For example, in Addis Ababa in 1982–83, 74% of the births were to women aged between 20 and 35 years (8).

Estimating the impact that avoiding risky early and late pregnancies might have on maternal mortality in any one place is complex and depends critically on a number of factors. These include the excess risk run by women in the so-called high-risk categories compared with other women, the number of births to such women expressed as a proportion of all births, and the effectiveness of contraceptives. Generally, the higher the excess risk (or the relative risk, as it is called) and the larger the proportion of births taking place to women in the high-risk categories, the greater the scope for reducing the overall maternal mortality rate.

Actual estimates vary. Calculations based on the Bangladesh figures cited above show that if the proportion of births among the high-risk age groups is eliminated, without a concomitant reduction in the number of births, then the maternal mortality rate will be reduced by only 9% (9, 10). However, preventing births to high-risk women altogether (and thereby also reducing fertility) would reduce the maternal mortality rate by 25%. The most probable effect of family planning on the maternal mortality rate, as distinct from its impact on the number of maternal deaths, probably lies somewhere between. (Estimates of the potential of family planning to reduce maternal deaths by both risk reduction and by avoiding unwanted births is discussed more fully below.)

Moreover, any realistic estimate of the scope for risk reduction must also take into account the fact of contraceptive failure. Even under the most favourable conditions, some women wishing to avoid pregnancy and using contraception do get pregnant.

## Reducing the absolute number of pregnancies

Family planning that is less narrowly focused and aims to provide services for all women of childbearing age is far more likely to result in a reduction in the number of maternal deaths. This is especially so where family planning succeeds in lowering fertility from a traditionally high level.

Lowering the total fertility rate (TFR)[1] reduces the **lifetime** risk for the individual woman even if the maternal mortality rate (the risk associated with each pregnancy) remains high: where families are traditionally large, women run a greater risk of dying as a result of pregnancy than women who traditionally have small families. Thus the average lifetime risk of pregnancy-related death for a woman in Africa is one in 25, compared with one in 38 in South Asia, one in 870 in East Asia, and one in 1750 in the developed world (see also Chapter 3).

According to UN estimates (*11*), TFRs range widely: 2.2–6.5 for Latin America and the Caribbean; 1.7–6.9 for Asia; 3.8–7.2 for the Eastern Mediteranean countries and North Africa, and 2.2–8.1 for sub-Saharan Africa. As can be seen from Table 9.1, the average TFR in the developing countries is twice that in the developed countries; that for Africa as a whole is three times as high.

A number of interesting factors have emerged from the many surveys of contraceptive use that have been carried out in

Table 9.1. Total fertility rates, by region

| Region | No. of women aged 15–49 (millions) 1985 | Total fertility rate 1980–85 |
|---|---|---|
| Developing countries | 892.3 | 4.1 |
| Africa | 125.3 | 6.3 |
| Asia and Oceania | 667.6 | 3.6 |
| East Asia | 294.1 | 2.4 |
| South Asia and Oceania | 373.5 | 4.6 |
| Latin America | 99.4 | 4.1 |
| Developed countries | 296.2 | 2.0 |
| World total | 1188.5 | 3.5 |

*Source*: United Nations (*11*).

---

[1] The *total fertility rate* is the number of children the average woman would have in her lifetime if she continued, at each age, to bear children at the same rate as do women today.

recent years. By questioning women about their pregnancy and childbearing history, researchers found that, in general, women who married at or after the age of 22 had, on average, 0.5 fewer children than those who married at 18 or 19 (*12*). Furthermore, the highest fertility is concentrated in different age bands in different parts of the world. In Colombia, Fiji, Malaysia, Paraguay, the Republic of Korea, Turkey and Thailand, for instance, most children are born to women between the ages of 20 and 29. The age band with the most concentrated childbearing is narrower than this (20–24) in such countries as Jamaica, Guyana, Panama and the Dominican Republic, and, as one would expect, tends to be wider (20–34) in countries where fertility is highest, such as Pakistan and some Eastern Mediterranean and North African countries.

Fertility levels are determined by the interaction of many different factors—social, cultural, economic, religious (see also Chapter 4). Each factor in turn affects, and is affected by, women's attitude to, knowledge of and practice of family planning. It is not yet possible to measure the effect of any single factor on fertility, or even to identify the exact mechanism by which this effect works. However, certain trends and relationships can be observed.

Education, for instance, is strongly related to fertility in most developing countries. Data from 38 countries relating to the late 1970s and early 1980s give an average fertility rate of 3.9 among women with 7 or more years of schooling compared with a rate of 6.9 among women with no schooling (*13*). The differential appears to be highest in Latin America (up to 5), and lowest in Africa (between 1 and 3). The latter observation is at least partly explained by the tradition of the extended family in which the support of children is a shared responsibility, and a large family does not necessarily represent a barrier to the educational or occupational advancement of the mother. The relationship between education and fertility is, however, not linear. Women with only a few years' schooling may in fact have more children than women with no schooling, chiefly because they will breast-feed their children for a shorter period and perhaps also because they no longer adhere to traditional patterns of postpartum abstinence.

In most countries—particularly in Latin America—there are marked differences between the urban and rural populations. In Honduras, for instance, while the TFR for the whole country in 1981 was 6.5, the average number of children born to urban women was 4.1 and among the rural population, 8.2. Similarly, in southern Brazil in 1981 the TFR was 3.3 in urban areas and 5.3 in rural areas. In Bangladesh, however, there was a difference of only 0.1 between urban and rural women (*13*).

The relationship between women's employment and fertility is particularly difficult to interpret. As a general rule women who work outside the home have fewer children, but it is rarely clear whether the lower number of children is a cause or result of the fact that they work. Besides, in the least developed countries, and where women's status is generally low, the difference in fertility levels between working women and non-working women is often insignificant (*14*) (see also Chapter 4). It has been observed, too, that among developing countries there are some, like Indonesia and the Philippines, with high fertility and a high proportion of women in the labour force, and others, like Chile and Sri Lanka, where the fertility rates are relatively low and so also is the proportion of working women.

The most important question as far as family planning and its potential for saving lives is concerned is: do women really want as many children as they are having? Evidence suggests that a considerable proportion of the high fertility observed in developing countries is unwanted.

The number of induced abortions is one measure of unwanted pregnancy; it has been estimated (*15*) that every year more than 40 million women take this course of action, or that between one-fifth and one-third of all pregnancies are terminated (see also Chapter 6).

Another measure is the information gathered by the World Fertility Surveys, in which women were questioned about their ideal family size. The surveys found a good deal of discrepancy between actual fertility and "wanted" fertility. In most Latin American countries, where the average family has 5 or 6 children, women said that the ideal family size was 2 or 3 children, i.e., about half the births are unwanted. In Asia the picture is more mixed. In some countries, such as Sri Lanka, Thailand and the Republic of Korea, wanted fertility rates, at around 2.6, are not very different from actual fertility rates which are 3.7, 3.9 and 2.6 respectively. In Bangladesh, however, actual fertility is over twice as high as desired. This is the case, too, in general in North Africa, but in sub-Saharan Africa the tendency is for married women to want as many children as they have, if not more (*16*).

It has been estimated that if women could have the number of children they desired and no more, the number of births would be reduced by an average of 35% (4.4 million) in Latin America, 33% (24.4 million) in Asia and 17% (4 million) in Africa.[1] The number of maternal deaths would fall by at least an equivalent proportion. Thus, for example, a reduction of 35% in fertility directly reduces the average woman's lifetime risk of dying from pregnancy-related causes by 35%, even though it does nothing to make pregnancy safer.

The independent contributions of fertility and maternal mortality risk are illustrated in Fig. 9.2. The height of the columns represents the lifetime risk of dying from pregnancy-related causes, which is a product of fertility (the left-hand axis) and the maternal mortality rate (the right-hand axis). For example, a woman living in Bangladesh, where the maternal mortality rate is about 700 per 100 000 and the total fertility rate is 6.2, has a lifetime chance of dying from pregnancy-related causes of 1 in 19. The diagram illustrates how her chances of dying could be reduced in one of two ways (or by a combination of the two). A reduction in fertility would enable her to step down towards the right. Lowering the risk associated with each pregnancy and childbirth, i.e., a reduction in the maternal mortality rate, would enable her to step down to the left. An even greater reduction could be effected if both fertility and mortality were to be reduced.

Another feature illustrated by Fig. 9.2 is the fact that the potential for risk reduction, or rather the most appropriate action to be taken under any given circumstances, depends to a great extent on the relative magnitudes of the two factors involved. Thus a lifetime risk of 1 in 31 can be caused by a TFR of 7 in combination with a maternal mortality rate of 300, or by a TFR of 3 in combination with a maternal mortality rate of 700. Clearly the scope for risk reduction through family planning is much greater in the first case than in the second.

---

[1] Maine, D. et al. *Prevention of maternal deaths in developing countries: program options and practical considerations.* Paper prepared for the International Safe Motherhood Conference, Nairobi, 10–13 February 1987.

Fig. 9.2. Lifetime risk of dying from pregnancy-related causes, according to fertility and prevailing maternal mortality rate.

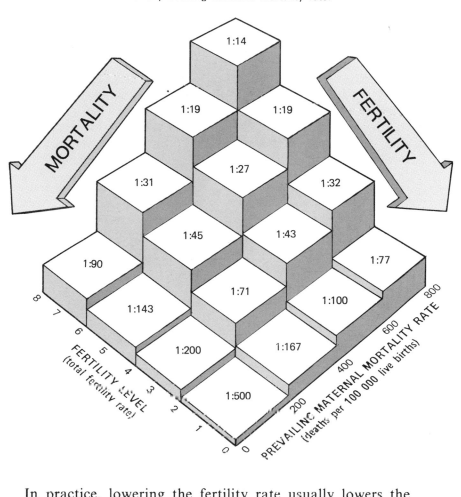

In practice, lowering the fertility rate usually lowers the lifetime risk of dying from pregnancy-related causes, and hence the total number of maternal deaths, more than proportionately, for a number of reasons. Firstly and most importantly, deaths from induced abortion are greatly reduced. Secondly, the very fact that a pregnancy is unwanted increases the risk to the mother, because women with unwanted pregnancies tend to neglect their health needs. An analysis of maternal deaths in Addis Ababa, for example, found that only about half of the women with unwanted pregnancies bothered to go for prenatal care, and those who did so tended to go to MCH clinics where the service was free, rather than to a hospital or private clinic. Furthermore, the women with unwanted pregnancies were least likely to deliver at hospital or with a trained attendant (8).

193

Lastly, the births that would be avoided if women were to have only their desired number of children would tend to be the higher risk births—the higher parity births to older women.

Thus, family planning enables women to bear children according to a relatively risk-free pattern and to avoid unwanted pregnancies, and in this way could make a considerable impact on the number of maternal deaths.

But this is pure hypothesis. It presupposes a vast increase in the spread of services, and a much higher degree of effectiveness than is the case in many of the programmes that exist already.

## "Unmet need" for family planning

According to the World Fertility Survey, less than half the married women who said they wanted no more children were using contraception. The discrepancy was most pronounced in Africa, where an average of only 23% of those who wanted no more children were using contraception, compared with 43% in Asia and 57% in Latin America (see Table 9.2).

Table 9.2. Women who want no more children and are using contraception (currently married women aged 15–44), selected countries

| Country or area | Percentage of women who want no more children | Percentage of those who want no more children who use contraception |
|---|---|---|
| *Africa* | | |
| Benin, 1981–82 | 6 | 25 |
| Botswana, 1984 | 30 | 35 |
| Côte d'Ivoire, 1980–81 | 4 | 9 |
| Ghana, 1979–80 | 10 | 19 |
| Kenya, 1977–78 | 15 | 16 |
| Lesotho, 1977 | 14 | 16 |
| Mauritania, 1981 | 10 | 2 |
| Nigeria, 1981–82 | 4 | 11 |
| Senegal | 7 | 2 |
| Sudan (north), 1978–79 | 16 | 12 |
| Zaire (Kinshasa), 1982–84 | 17 | 38 |
| Zimbabwe, 1984 | 20 | 48 |

## Table 9.2 (continued)

| Country or area | Percentage of women who want no more children | Percentage of those who want no more children who use contraception |
|---|---|---|
| **Asia and the Pacific** | | |
| Bangladesh, 1979–80 | 45 | 22 |
| Fiji, 1974 | 48 | 61 |
| Indonesia (Java and Bali), 1976 | 37 | 47 |
| Indonesia (Jakarta), 1983 | 59 | 54 |
| Malaysia (peninsular), 1974 | 43 | 48 |
| Nepal, 1981 | 36 | 16 |
| Pakistan, 1975 | 41 | 12 |
| Philippines, 1978 | 53 | 51 |
| Republic of Korea, 1979 | 74 | 69 |
| Sri Lanka, 1982 | 64 | 69 |
| Thailand, 1981 | 65 | 69 |
| **Latin America and the Caribbean** | | |
| Barbados, 1980–81 | 48 | 56 |
| Bolivia, 1983 | 73 | 24 |
| Brazil | | |
| Amazonas (urban), 1982 | 62 | 69 |
| North-east region, 1980 | 57 | 48 |
| Piaui, 1979 | 69 | 36 |
| Piaui, 1982 | 56 | 48 |
| São Paulo, 1978 | 62 | 77 |
| Southern region, 1981 | 49 | 80 |
| Colombia, 1980 | 64 | 56 |
| Costa Rica, 1981 | 51 | 72 |
| Dominican Republic, 1983 | 72 | 58 |
| Ecuador, 1979 | 55 | 44 |
| El Salvador, 1978 | 46 | 46 |
| Guatemala, 1983 | 38 | 45 |
| Guyana, 1975 | 57 | 43 |
| Haiti, 1983 | 48 | 10 |
| Honduras, 1981 | 57 | 29 |
| Jamaica, 1983 | 54 | 57 |
| Mexico, 1978 | 64 | 49 |
| Paraguay, 1979 | 29 | 45 |
| Peru, 1981 | 73 | 45 |
| Trinidad and Tobago, 1977 | 52 | 64 |
| Venezuela, 1977 | 55 | 57 |
| **North Africa and Eastern Mediterranean** | | |
| Egypt, 1980 | 52 | 41 |
| Jordan, 1983 | 42 | 38 |
| Morocco, 1979–80 | 39 | 43 |
| Syrian Arab Republic, 1978 | 34 | 41 |
| Tunisia, 1983 | 63 | 53 |
| Yemen Arab Republic, 1979 | 18 | 4 |

Interestingly, Table 9.2 shows that where contraceptive use to stop childbearing is weakest, the proportion of women who say they want no more children also tends to be lowest, which suggests that social support is an important part of the equation.

The gap highlighted by the World Fertility Survey between women's expressed desire to stop childbearing and their effective action to achieve this goal is a measure of the "unmet need" for family planning. But it is only a partial measure, for it does not take account of the women who want to space births but are not using contraception, or of sexually active unmarried women who want to avoid pregnancy or space births but who are also not using contraception.

The importance of each of the various categories will depend on the fertility patterns and sexual mores of the particular society. Thus, in sub-Saharan Africa, where the desire for many children is generally strong, the greatest need for contraception is likely to be for birth spacing rather than for limiting childbearing, while in a country like Jamaica, where sexual activity outside marriage is common and relatively socially acceptable, the family planning needs of unmarried women are particularly significant (*17*). In both of these cases the WFS data would give a distorted picture of unmet need if they were taken as the sole measure. Fig. 9.3 shows the

Fig. 9.3. Percentage of women who want more children and who are using temporary contraception, selected countries, late 1970s

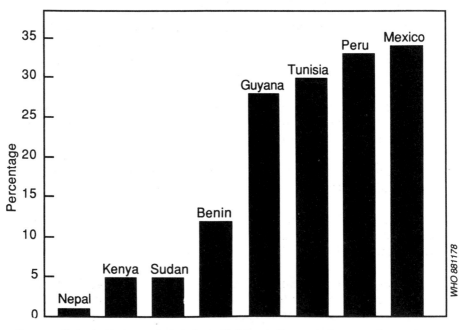

*Source*: United Nations. Population Division. *Contraceptive practice: selected findings from the World Fertility Survey data.* Document ESA/P/WP/93, 1986.

proportion of women in some selected countries who use contraception for spacing births.

The reasons that women who want to control their fertility do not use contraception fall into two main categories:

(a) Lack of services: coverage is inadequate and some people are thereby denied the opportunity to practise modern contraception.

(b) Inappropriate services: the services that are available are not suited to people's needs.

## Lack of services

As recently as the early 1960s the taboo surrounding family planning was such that it was never included on the agenda of any United Nations body. Though this antipathy at the international level has been overcome to the extent that family planning is now considered a basic human right, individual countries and peoples have different degrees of commitment to it. Some countries are pronatalist and therefore discourage the use of contraception. This was the case in Greece until 1980 (18). Other countries, such as Ireland, may oppose it on religious grounds, while for the French-speaking countries of sub-Saharan Africa poor commitment to family planning services is a legacy of the colonial period and the French anti-contraception law of 1920, which was not liberalized in France itself until 1967 (19). In Saudi Arabia, too, contraceptives have been banned.

In some cases people do not have access to family planning services because they live in remote places beyond the reach of modern services. But even where physical isolation is not a problem, there are some groups that remain difficult to reach, highlighting the fact that the provision of services is a matter of information as well as supplies.

Access to family planning implies familiarity with the subject of contraception first and foremost, followed by knowledge of where the service can be obtained.

The World Fertility Surveys and the Contraceptive Prevalence Surveys revealed that there are vast numbers of people with no knowledge at all of modern contraceptive methods. The proportion of currently married women aged 15–44 who knew of at least one modern method ranged from only 6% in

Mauritania to 100% in Fiji. The level of knowledge was generally low in sub-Saharan Africa (between 6% and 60%), with some notable exceptions such as Botswana (80%), Kenya (89%), and Zimbàbwe (89%) and generally high in all other regions (between 75% and 100%) except in Bolivia (51%), Nepal (52%) and the Yemen Arab Republic (24%) (14).

At least a quarter of the women in Bangladesh, Barbados, Dominican Republic, Honduras, and Indonesia did not know of any source of contraceptive supplies, while the proportion amounted to 85% in Nepal and 93% in Somalia. Only in Paraguay, Tobago, and Venezuela was the proportion of "don't knows" less than 10% (14).

Rural people are, as a general rule, more difficult to reach with information about family planning, but their access to services is also likely to be more restricted than that of urban people because of greater distance from clinics and sources of supply. A study of contraceptive use in Jendouba province, Tunisia—a region of predominantly rural and widely scattered inhabitants—found that the level among rural women was only 50% of that found among urban women, and the fact that they needed to travel to hospital or clinic-based facilities in the cities explained much of the discrepancy. Most of the women had to use public transport or walk, and many said they did not know exactly where to go for supplies (20).

Frequently there are other, more subtle, barriers. For instance, in some countries oral contraceptives are available only on prescription, and the extra contact with health or family planning staff necessary to obtain supplies may render it impractical for some women.

Experience shows that it is often those in most need of family planning, whether in the cities or the countryside, who are most difficult to reach: the poor and underprivileged who may be unable to support large families. In Guatemala, for instance, the Contraceptive Prevalence Survey of 1978 revealed that Indian groups had particularly low levels of contraceptive use, so a special effort was made through radio information in Indian dialects and by training community members as promoters (14).

In many countries unmarried women are denied their right to family planning, usually on moral grounds. But the evidence shows that this rarely prevents sexual activity among unmarried people; it simply leaves large numbers of women vulnerable to unwanted pregnancy.

## Inappropriate services

Even where logistic problems have been more or less solved, many family planning programmes achieve only a fraction of their full potential simply because they do not meet the needs of their "customers", for a variety of reasons.

A common problem is that family planning is often targeted at the female users of contraceptives, ignoring the fact that women may have little personal choice in such matters. In many societies, decisions—even about childbearing—are taken by the men, or even by the elders of a family clan (see Chapter 4). In Zaire, for instance, where traditionally the extended family takes collective responsibility for the support of children, it is the wife's brothers (in matrilineal groups) or the husband's father and brothers (in patrilineal groups) who decide on matters of childbearing (*21*). If a family planning programme fails to address the real decision-makers and to enlist the support of community leaders, it will waste a good deal of effort.

So, too, a programme that fails to understand the cultural beliefs and practices of its customers may waste effort by providing contraceptives that are not widely acceptable, or by failing to give adequate information to allay fears and superstitions.

Three of the most important contraceptive methods—the pill, the intrauterine device (IUD) and injectable contraceptives—all disrupt menstruation to a greater or lesser degree, and this is likely to be an important drawback in cultures that impose restrictions on menstruating women. A WHO study of 14 cultural groups in ten different countries found some kind of behavioural restriction associated with menstruation in every one. These included prohibition of sexual intercourse, hair washing, bathing, washing clothes, praying and visiting newly delivered women (*22*).

Conversely, contraceptives that inhibit the menstrual flow find disfavour with other family planning users: 50% of women surveyed in the Republic of Korea and 91% in Pakistan expressed themselves opposed to such methods on grounds of health, as well as for the reason that they felt reassured in their femininity, potential fertility, or avoidance of pregnancy by the arrival of their regular period (22).

Fears that contraceptives can cause serious disease, get lost in the body, or affect sexuality are also fairly widespread, and exert a strong influence, however misguided they may be.

Bodily inhibitions can also affect acceptance of contraceptives. Where there are taboos or inhibitions against women manipulating their genitals, diaphragms, foams and jellies will be distasteful. Furthermore, women may be reluctant to attend clinics where they are worried about lack of privacy, being questioned about very personal matters, and perhaps being attended by a male member of staff. Lack of privacy can bring problems at home too. Where women live under crowded conditions they may find it difficult to store contraceptives or dispose of them without others knowing.

A major influence on contraceptive use is, of course, religion. The Roman Catholic church's opposition to intercourse without the possibility of procreation can have a profound effect on its followers. Neither Islam nor Hinduism has a spiritual basis for opposition to family planning. Nevertheless, some individual religious leaders are personally antipathetic and may influence their followers. Jewish law is particularly opposed to sterilization because it is considered to be surgical impairment of the reproductive organs and "deliberate interference with the natural practice of generation" (23).

The examples touched upon here show that sensitivity to the social and cultural climate is vital if family planning is to be effective. They also indicate that giving people as wide a choice of contraceptive methods as possible greatly enhances the prospects of success.

## The unmet needs of adolescents

Adolescents deserve special consideration because, as a group, they are the most ill-served of all by family planning programmes, and because their needs in many respects are peculiar to their age and social standing.

Adolescents are also a large and growing proportion of the population, amounting to 23% of the total population of developing countries in 1985. The absolute number of females aged 15–19 is expected to triple in Africa by the year 2020,

and to increase by 50% in Latin America by the same time
(*24*).

From the point of view of family planning, adolescents can
be divided into two categories—those who are married and
those who are single (see Chapter 4 for the incidence of
adolescent marriage).

Surveys have shown that, among married adolescents in
developing countries, contraceptive use is generally extremely
low. In Africa, the proportion using contraceptives ranges
from 1% to 6.5%, with Tunisia being an exception at over
10%; in Asia the proportion ranges from under 5% in
Bangladesh to 28% in Sri Lanka and 29% in Thailand. In
Latin America, prevalence of contraceptive use among
married adolescents is above 20% in the majority of
countries, with El Salvador and Honduras being exceptions
at 8% (*24*).

These low levels are not surprising since the same social
conditions that favour very early marriage also favour early
childbearing (see Chapter 4). It is important that family
planning workers make an effort to reach this special group
with education, information and services because of the
particularly high risks to mother and child posed by
adolescent pregnancy and childbirth.

It is generally recognized that raising the age of marriage is
one of the most effective ways of discouraging very early
motherhood. This measure is also likely to increase contraceptive acceptance among adolescent wives by indicating
social approval of later childbearing.

As far as unmarried adolescents are concerned, the issue of
family planning is a particularly sensitive one because of its
moral overtones. By international convention[1] the "right" to
adequate education, information and services for all
individuals and couples to enable them to take personal
responsibility for their own fertility covers adolescents as
well. Yet there is a widespread fear that providing such
services to young people outside the context of marriage will
encourage promiscuity. In some countries this moral conflict

---

[1] First expressed as a resolution at the UN Conference on Human Rights in
Teheran in 1968, reaffirmed in 1974 by the UN Population Conference in Bucharest,
and again in 1984 at the International Population Conference in Mexico City.

has not been resolved, with the result that, for many adolescents, the path of personal development is strewn with unnecessary hazards.

Though exact figures are impossible to ascertain, there is evidence that sexual activity among unmarried adolescents is increasingly common. Data from Jamaica's largest maternity hospital in Kingston for 1976–77, for example, showed that nearly one-third of births were to adolescents, most of whom were schoolgirls (17). In Nigeria, too, there is evidence of this phenomenon: a survey of 45 schools found that only 12 had been unaffected by pregnancy among their young pupils (25), while a 1982 survey of 240 high school students found that 43% of the females were sexually experienced (24).

Abortion is another indication of sexual activity among unmarried adolescents, and in sub-Saharan Africa it is, at present, more common among young, unmarried urban women than among women of any other status. Studies in several Latin American cities in 1968–71 found that the rate of abortion among adolescents, while lower than the rate among older women at the time, was rising faster than in any other group. And in countries where abortion is legal the rate among adolescents rose steadily throughout the 1970s (24).

Though premarital sexual activity appears to be widespread in many parts of the world, disapproval or ambivalence on the part of some governments towards the whole question of adolescent sexuality means that many young people are extremely ill-prepared. Though some developing countries—notably the Philippines and Costa Rica—are strongly committed to sex education, this is absent from the curriculum in the majority of other developing countries. Sometimes this is because no statutory provision has been made for sex education and it has been ignored (as in Bangladesh and much of sub-Saharan Africa), and sometimes because it has been actively legislated against (as in many French-speaking African countries). Sometimes general sex education is permitted, while specific information on contraception is prohibited (24).

Family planning programmes that aim to reach young people have to take account of their access to information and its reliability. They also have to recognize a wide range of constraints against unmarried women—and particularly those who are still legally "minors"—using family planning services.

## Contraceptive methods

According to United Nations estimates (*11*), the level of contraceptive use among married or cohabiting couples with the woman in the reproductive age group is 51% for the world as a whole. This reflects a rapid rate of increase; in the mid-1960s the rate was under 10%. Prevalence in developing countries has reached 45%: 74% in East Asia, 54% in Latin America, 33% in South Asia and 14% in Africa.

In developing areas, contraceptive prevalence ranges from as low as 1% of couples in Mauritania and Yemen to 70–75% in China, Hong Kong, Mauritius, Puerto Rico, the Republic of Korea and Singapore. In the developed countries the range is narrower; prevalence is at least 50% in all countries and in most it is over 70%.

Contraceptive prevalence is still very low, with no sign of substantial change, in most of Africa south of the Sahara and in parts of Asia. However, there is evidence of an increase in some countries where use levels had been low and static until recently, including Bangladesh, Nepal and Pakistan.

The prevalence of the main methods is summarized below and in Fig. 9.4:

female sterilization—154 million couples;
male sterilization—60 million couples;
intrauterine device—110 million couples;
oral contraceptives—95 million couples;
condom—59 million couples;
injectables, female barrier methods, or spermicides—
11 million couples.

An estimated 120 million couples were using abstinence, withdrawal or another "traditional" form of contraception. In addition to these, around 40–50 million women seek abortion every year for unwanted pregnancy, of which around 50% might be the result of contraceptive failure.

## Switching and discontinuation

Close observation reveals that there is a good deal of inconsistency in the use of contraceptives. It is quite common,

Fig. 9.4. Use of contraceptives throughout the world

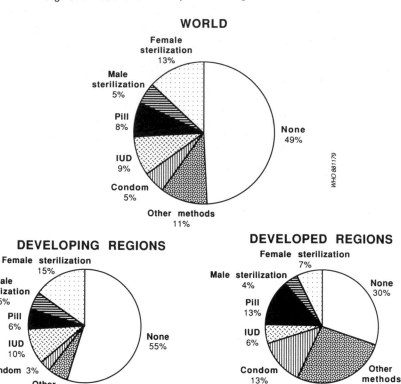

Source: United Nations (11).

for instance, for people to change methods or to lapse altogether in their use within a year or so. The World Fertility Survey data give a rough indication of the extent of method-switching and/or discontinuation. For all regions of the developing world covered by the survey the numbers of people using a particular method as a percentage of those who had ever used that same method were:

38% for the pill;

23% for condoms;

27% for injectables;

17% for female barrier methods;

44% for IUD.

The data do not reveal what proportion of those who had stopped using one particular method had switched to another and what proportion had discontinued altogether, but it is thought to be around 50% for each category.

Continuation rates appear to be influenced by the level of development in a country and by the strength of the family planning programme. Thus the World Fertility Survey found that where the level of development was high. and the family planning effort strong, continuation rates were also likely to be high, and vice versa.

Apart from interruptions in supplies or services, the reasons for discontinuation of contraception included:

(a) unacceptable side-effects (real or imagined) and limited choice of alternatives;

(b) inconvenience of method;

(c) interference with intercourse;

(d) loss of personal motivation, perhaps aggravated by low social support for family planning.

It is reasonable to expect that contraceptive users will change methods from time to time according to their life circumstances and family planning needs. A young woman with no family might, for instance, choose the pill to postpone childbearing, the IUD to space births later on, and sterilization when she wants no more children. Or couples may need to try several different methods in succession before finding one that suits them. In any case, method switching and lapses of contraceptive use highlight the need for as wide a choice of methods as possible in a family planning programme if it is to achieve maximum coverage and effectiveness.

## Risks and benefits

Risk assessment can be a controversial issue. Some people believe that the only relevant measure of contraceptive safety is the absolute risk associated with a method (i.e., the risk of morbidity or death per 1000 users). However, it is widely agreed that the health risk of a contraceptive method is more meaningful when compared with the risk of pregnancy and childbirth. From the latter viewpoint the health risks of a particular contraceptive method will loom largest where pregnancy and childbirth pose little threat to a woman, and appear least significant where childbearing is particularly hazardous (Fig. 9.5). Different countries might therefore be expected to have different views on the acceptability of some contraceptive methods.

A thorough analysis of risk should also take account of the failure rate of a method (see Fig. 9.6) and therefore the risk

Fig. 9.5. Estimated annual deaths resulting from pregnancy, childbirth, abortion, contraceptive use and unintended pregnancy following contraceptive failure

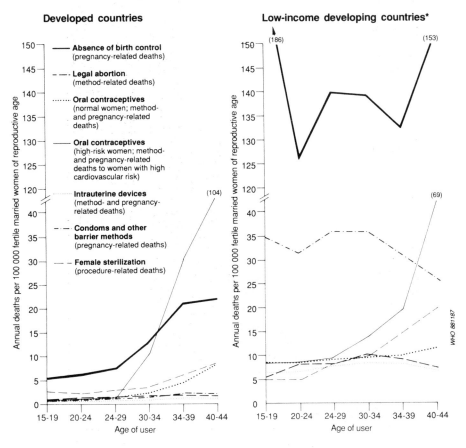

* Countries with per capita incomes of less than US$410 and with average maternal mortality rates of about 350 deaths per 100 000 live births.

Notes: Maternal death estimates assume lower use-effectiveness rates in developing countries for all methods except the IUD.
The risk of death related to sterilization is a one-time risk. Data that reflect estimated deaths per 100 000 procedures rather than per 100 000 women overstate relative risks over time compared to other methods.

*Source*: Population Crisis Committee (*28*).

Fig. 9.6. Estimated range of failure rates for major contraceptive methods

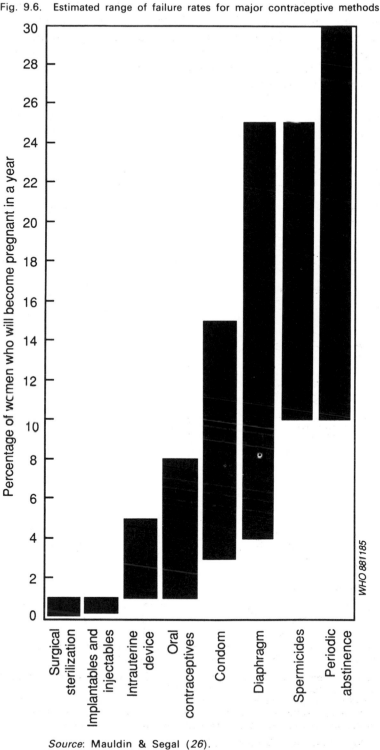

WHO 881185

*Source*: Mauldin & Segal (*26*).

associated with accidental pregnancy, including abortion as a possible response. Thus, if mortality is the most important consideration, in a developing country with a high maternal mortality rate (indicating high obstetric risk) and no legal abortion, the lowest risk would be found in using the most reliable contraceptive method. Conversely, in a developed country with very low maternal mortality (indicating minimal obstetric risk) and legal abortion, the lowest risk would be found in using the safest, but relatively unreliable, contraceptive method such as the condom or diaphragm, with abortion as a backup in case of failure.

As a general rule, any modern method of contraception is safer than pregnancy or childbirth for women anywhere in the world, with the exception of the pill for high-risk women over 39 in developed countries (see Fig. 9.5). However, for each individual woman the balance of risks between contraception and pregnancy will be different, and will depend on such factors as age, parity, nutritional and health status, as well as on living conditions, access to medical care and, of course, the method of contraception chosen.

Furthermore, a component of the "risk equation" that is often overlooked is the fact that a number of the modern methods of contraception have additional, non-contraceptive health benefits. Thus, hormonal contraceptives reduce the amount of blood loss at menstruation and hence reduce the risk of anaemia. They have also been shown to be protective against certain forms of cancer—of the ovaries and of the endometrium (the lining of the uterus) (27)—and to reduce the risk of pelvic infections (28).

## The concept of "reproductive mortality"

In order to encompass both the risk of pregnancy and childbirth and the risk associated with trying to avoid pregnancy, the concept of "reproductive mortality" has been developed, which gives a more holistic view of a woman's chances of dying during her fertile years. This concept is important in calculating the potential of a family planning programme for saving lives. The need for such a measure is clearest in developed countries, where pregnancy and childbirth entail low risk, since the maternal mortality figures alone will give only a partial view of deaths related to reproduction. For example, in the United States of America in 1975 only 53% of reproductive deaths were pregnancy-related (i.e., maternal deaths) while virtually all the rest (45%) were related to oral contraceptive use (29). In contrast, in Menoufia, Egypt, in 1981–83 and in Bali, Indonesia, in 1980–82, 98% of reproductive mortality was pregnancy-related (30).

## What does the future hold?

There are a number of constraints on the development of new contraceptive methods. First, there is a lack of investment. In 1984 the combined total expenditure by governments, international agencies, pharmaceutical companies and private research institutions was around US$ 175 million—less in real terms than a decade earlier (28).

Secondly, the investment in time and money necessary to bring a new contraceptive on to the market—ranging typically from 5 to 20 years and $ 20 million to $ 70 million, partly because of the extremely strict testing requirements—makes research in this field unattractive to pharmaceutical companies, particularly as a patent for a new product may expire before it even reaches the marketplace.

China, India, Mexico, Singapore and Thailand are becoming increasingly important as centres of research, and the WHO Special Programme of Research, Development and Research Training in Human Reproduction involves an international network of 45 research centres in 30 different countries. However, research and development of contraceptives still take place predominantly in the developed countries, which has a number of drawbacks for developing countries. Risk-benefit and cost-effectiveness analyses based on conditions in developed countries may not be widely relevant to developing countries.

However, despite such constraints and the shortage of funds, several new methods are emerging from research supported by the WHO Special Programme and others that should have wide cross-cultural appeal. These include:

(a) Once-a-month injectable contraceptives containing an estrogen as well as a progestogen. Their advantage over progestogen-only methods is that they permit regular menstrual bleeding episodes; moreover, the injectables are virtually 100% effective.

(*b*) Vaginal rings, which slowly release contraceptive hormones. They can be inserted by the user herself. This method has the advantage over the IUD, injectables and implants that it is the only long-acting method to be under the direct control of the woman herself. A 3-month ring may be available in some countries by 1990.

(*c*) Slow-release microspheres consisting of hormone in a soluble substance (a polymer carrier) which, after injection, dissolves and releases hormone at a given rate. The first contraceptive of this type delivers norethisterone over a period of 3 months (*31*).

(*d*) A "menstrual inducer" for use when the menstrual period is late. Anti-progestins offer a new approach to menses induction by medical means, through oral administration. A combination of anti-progestin and prostaglandin will have the advantage of higher effectiveness than the older methods, especially when the menstrual period has been delayed for a longer time.

(*e*) A contraceptive vaccine for women which would give reversible long-term protection against pregnancy. The vaccine is based on the pregnancy hormone chorionic gonadotrophin. It is expected to offer protection for up to two years.

(*f*) Contraceptives for men, both hormonal and non-hormonal. Lack of development in this field till now largely reflects the fact that, for biological reasons, the control of male fertility by pharmacological methods is proving to be much more difficult than the control of female fertility.

(*g*) Reliable indicators of ovulation to help those who wish to practise natural family planning—or periodic abstinence—to do so effectively.

## Design and delivery of services

As the section on inappropriate services indicated, a successful family planning programme needs to understand the factors within society that influence decisions about childbearing and to be very sensitive to the needs and circumstances of the particular community that it serves. Sometimes this means recognizing that family planning is not perceived as a priority by the targeted population.

Lessons from the field indicate that family planning that forms part of an integrated programme of development designed to meet people's most pressing needs is more readily accepted than a family planning programme with a more limited focus on its own goals.

At the Alma-Ata Conference in 1978, family planning was identified as one of the components of primary health care, and there are indeed many places where it is delivered through the health services network. This makes sense in view of the fact that several contraceptive methods—such as the IUD, sterilization, and sometimes the pill—require medical intervention. MCH services, prenatal and postnatal clinics, which bring women into contact with the health services, can provide ideal opportunities for contraceptive counselling. Furthermore, identifying family planning with health can help to make it more acceptable politically, especially where there is widespread suspicion of population policies.

However, integrated programmes that include family planning need not necessarily revolve around health care. Since 1976 the International Planned Parenthood Federation (IPPF) has been supporting a wide range of programmes under its Planned Parenthood and Women's Development (PPWD) scheme, begun in recognition of the close connection between fertility and women's status (17).

One such project, started in 1977, has been assisting a very poor and socially deprived ethnic minority group in Costa Rica to develop marketable skills so that they can earn a living. The scheme includes craft training and the setting up of workshops and business cooperatives, which also provide a focal point for educational activities. These include responsible parenthood and sex education as well as family planning. Very gradually, as the women's horizons open up, family planning becomes a relevant issue.

Another project supported under the PPWD scheme works with adolescents in Jamaica who have been forced by pregnancy to drop out of school before they have finished their education or acquired the skills needed to support themselves properly. A centre offers these girls a chance to continue their education and undertake vocational training. One of the most important elements in rebuilding self-esteem is the mutual support and encouragement that the girls give to one another. Because there is resistance to family planning generally—fostered by extreme ignorance of sex and contraception among the girls and tacit social acceptance of young men who father illegitimate children—the curriculum at the centre includes education and counselling related to sex and family planning. In an effort to promote responsible parenthood, the centre also tries to involve young men in its activities.

There are PPWD programmes in many countries. Each is tailored to the special needs of a particular community and is generally intended to reach the very poorest people. One of the main lessons learned over the years has been the need for careful preliminary planning and for realism—both in the goals set and in the time needed to show results.

Establishing a network for the delivery of family planning and for keeping up supplies—particularly to remote rural communities—presents major problems in many developing countries. One answer to this has been the development of the community-based delivery (CBD) system whereby local people, after a brief training, are employed to provide certain family planning services to their own communities, either door-to-door or from a convenient local depot.

Essentially, CBD improves access by overcoming:

— geographical barriers;

— cost barriers (some distributors charge a small fee, some nothing);

— cultural and communication barriers;

— bureaucratic barriers (it minimizes reliance on clinics and professional medical personnel, thereby cutting down on waiting time and paperwork).

However CBD has one obvious limitation. Experience shows that wide choice is necessary for a high level of contraceptive acceptance, yet CBD is only suitable for contraceptive methods that are safe and easy to supply and require no medical intervention. Furthermore, where demand for family planning services is high, there may be a tendency to burden the untrained staff with responsibilities beyond their capability. This is likely to be a particular problem where family planning is combined with other services, such as the distribution of rehydration salts or malaria therapy.

When CBD started in the early 1970s it was considered a radical idea, but it is now widely accepted and operating in at least 40 countries (*32*). In 1978–79 one CBD project in Bangladesh in which pills, condoms, foaming tablets and injectables were distributed, achieved an increase of 27% in acceptance of contraceptives by married women of reproductive age. In Indonesia a CBD project distributing pills, condoms and injectables achieved an increase of 37% between 1978 and 1981.

Another delivery system that attempts to overcome logistic problems is social marketing. This was built on the recognition that manufacturers of consumer goods manage to get their products into the most remote village stores often well beyond the reach of modern government services.

Social marketing uses the commercial distribution network to provide contraceptives at subsidized prices in village stores. Furthermore it uses advertising in the mass media to promote them like any other commercial product. Convenience is the major advantage but, as with CBD, this method of delivery is only suitable for a limited range of contraceptives.

Mexico has a particularly dynamic social marketing organization called Profam which sells contraceptives— predominantly condoms—through foodstores and pharmacies across the country. Profam has predicted that it will eventually reach around 80% of Mexico's population (*33*).

These are just some examples of how family planning can be made more accessible to people. They all share the basic aim of giving individuals and couples the wherewithal to control their own fertility according to their own wishes and interests, rather than according to some demographic master plan. This orientation is crucial to success for, as Dr Halfdan Mahler, then Director-General of WHO, observed at the 1984 Population Conference in Mexico City (*34*): "Past attempts, divorced from development, to force measures of fertility control on abstract 'populations' gave rise only to resentment, resistance and rejection."

## Infertility

One important aspect of family planning programmes that has not yet been mentioned is their relevance to couples who are infertile. As Chapters 4, 6 and 7 have shown, infertility is a common phenomenon in some parts of the developing world; it can cause intense personal misery and, in cultures where motherhood is the only acceptable role for women, this can be compounded by ridicule and social isolation.

To a large extent the treatment of infertility draws on the same specialized knowledge and uses the same technology as the control of fertility (*35*). Family planning programmes should therefore provide counselling, and treatment where possible, for this condition. Discussion of the possible causes of infertility should also be included in sex education.

## The impact of family planning on child health

Another aspect of family planning that deserves mention is the effect that it has on the health of children. Though many different patterns have been observed, as a general rule the factors that put mothers at special risk also pose an increased risk to their children. Thus infants born to very young mothers or to mothers over 35 years, infants born at close intervals, and those of birth order number four or higher, are at greater risk of death or long-term ill health than others.

Taking the various risk factors in isolation, many studies indicate that birth spacing has more impact on infant health than either maternal age or birth order. In a 29-country study, infant mortality among those born after an interval of less than 2 years was on average 1.8 times higher than among those born after an interval of 2–4 years (*36*).

A study in the Punjab, India, found that the mortality rate for infants born after an interval of less than 11 months was as high as 206 per 1000, compared with rates of 132 per 1000 for those born after an interval of 24–35 months and 108 per 1000 for those born after an interval of 48 months or more (*35*).

Evidence suggests that short birth intervals affect the survival prospects of the preceding child also. A study in Pakistan, for example, found that a child was 1.4 times more likely to die before the age of two years if it was followed by a sibling within 18 months than if the interval was longer than this (*36*). The picture is extremely complex, but it is thought that early weaning plays a large part in undermining the health of the child whose birth is followed quickly by another pregnancy.

The increased risk of infant mortality associated with the age of the mother is generally most pronounced at the beginning of the childbearing spectrum. A study in northern Nigeria, for instance, found that one in five infants of mothers under the age of 16 died in the perinatal period—a rate 2.5 times higher than that for infants born to mothers aged 20–24 years (37).

As this brief discussion indicates, maternal and child survival are intimately related, and family planning that enhances the prospects of the mother also enhances the prospects of the infant. Furthermore, in the long term, child health and family planning are mutually reinforcing, for people are more ready to accept the idea of family planning if they are confident that their children will survive.

## Conclusion

Though the primary purpose of a family planning programme should be to give people the power to choose for themselves the number and timing of their children, it does, at the same time, serve the purpose of health planners by helping to reduce the risk of childbearing and to save lives.

However, in the battle against high levels of maternal mortality, family planning should never be seen as a substitute for obstetric care. This is a temptation where the health budget is limited and choices have to be made, because it is very much easier to achieve good coverage with family planning than with obstetric care. But it is morally unacceptable, for while a family planning service may reduce the number of women at risk of dying from pregnancy, it does nothing to reduce the risk for those who do become pregnant.

In the final analysis, the role of family planning in combating maternal mortality is to help create healthy conditions for childbearing, and to reduce the risk of pregnancy-related death for individual women. It is just one part of the complex answer to a complex problem.

## References

1. ECKHOLM, E. & NEWLAND, K. *Health: the family planning factor.* Washington, DC, Worldwatch Institute, 1977.
2. SAI, F. T. Family planning and maternal health care: a common goal. *World health forum*, 7(4): 315–340 (1986).

3. CHEN, L. C. ET AL. Maternal mortality in rural Bangladesh. *Studies in family planning*, **5**(11): 334–341 (1974).

4. WRIGHT, N. H. Thailand: estimates of the potential impact of family planning on maternal and infant mortality. *Journal of the Medical Association of Thailand*, **58**(4): 204–210 (1975).

5. NORTMAN, D. Parental age as a factor in child development. *Reports on population/family planning*, **16**: 1–52 (1974).

6. UNITED NATIONS. *Demographic indicators of countries: estimates and projections as assessed in 1980*. New York, Population Division, Department of International Economic and Social Affairs, 1982.

7. WALKER, G. J. ET AL. Maternal mortality in Jamaica. *Lancet*, **1**(8479): 486–488 (1986).

8. KWAST, B. E. ET AL. *Report on maternal health in Addis Ababa*. Addis Ababa, Swedish Save the Children Federation, 1984.

9. FORTNEY, J. A. The importance of family planning in reducing maternal mortality. *Studies in family planning*, **18**(2): 109–114 (1987).

10. TRUSSEL, J. & PEBLEY, A. R. The potential impact of changes in fertility on infant, child and maternal mortality. *Studies in family planning*, **15**(6): 267–279 (1984).

11. UNITED NATIONS. *World contraceptive use, 1987. Data sheet.* New York, Population Division, Department of International Economic and Social Affairs, 1987.

12. LIGHTBOURNE, R. ET AL. The World Fertility Survey: charting global childbearing. *Population bulletin*, **37**(1): 1–54 (1982).

13. UNITED NATIONS. *Fertility behaviour in the context of development. Evidence from the World Fertility Survey.* New York, Department of Economic and Social Affairs, 1987 (Population Studies No. 100).

14. LONDON, K. A. ET AL. Fertility and family planning surveys: an update. *Population reports*, Series M, **8**, 290–348 (1985).

15. TIETZE, C. & HENSHAW, S. K. *Induced abortion. A world review, 1986.* 6th ed. New York, Alan Guttmacher Institute, 1986.

16. LIGHTBOURNE, R. E. & MACDONALD, A. L. *Family size preferences.* Voorburg, Netherlands, International Statistical Institute and World Fertility Survey, 1982 (WFS comparative Studies No. 14).

17. INTERNATIONAL PLANNED PARENTHOOD FEDERATION. *Planned parenthood and women's development.* London, 1982.

18. LOVEL, H. & BAKOULA, C. Lack of family planning leading to induced abortion in rural Greece. *IPPF medical bulletin*, **19**(3): 1 (1985).

19. GIRARD, A. Pronatalist policies in Eastern Europe and France. *Draper Fund report*, **12**: 6–7 (1983).

20. MAGUIRE, E. ET AL. The delivery and use of contraceptive services in rural Tunisia. *International family planning perspectives*, **8**(3): 96–115 (1982).

21. KAYEMBE, T. B. Traditional structures clash with new imperatives. *Draper Fund report*, **12**: 3–5 (1983).

22. WHO SPECIAL PROGRAMME OF RESEARCH, DEVELOPMENT AND RESEARCH TRAINING IN HUMAN REPRODUCTION. A cross-cultural study of menstruation: implications for contraceptive development and use. *Studies in family planning*, **12**(1): 3–16 (1981).

23. GALLI, N. ET AL. Health education and sensitivity to cultural, religious and ethnic beliefs. *Journal of school health*, **57**(5): 177–180 (1987).

24. SENDEROWITZ, J. & PAXMAN, J. M. Adolescent fertility: worldwide concerns. *Population bulletin*, **40**(2): 1–51 (1985).

25. AKINGBA, J. B. Abortion, maternity and other health problems in Nigeria. *Nigerian medical journal,* **7**(4): 465–471 (1977).

26. MAULDIN, W. P. & SEGAL, S. J. *Prevalence of contraceptive use in developing countries. A chart book.* New York, Rockefeller Foundation, 1986.

27. HOLCK, S. Cancer and the pill. *World health*, November 1987.

28. POPULATION CRISIS COMMITTEE. Issues in contraceptive development. *Population*, No. 15 (May 1985).

29. SACHS, B. P. ET AL. Reproductive mortality in the United States. *Journal of the American Medical Association*, **247**(20): 2789–2792 (1982).

30. FORTNEY, J. A. ET AL. Reproductive mortality in two developing countries. *American journal of public health*, **76**(2): 134–136 (1986).

31. HALL, P. E. Quest for an ideal. *World health*, November 1987.

32. KOLS, A. J. ET AL. Community-based health and family planning. *Population reports*, Series L, No. 3: 111 (1982).

33. ROWLEY, J. Profam. Selling in the supermarket. *People*, **11**(3): (1984)

34. MAHLER, H. Family planning in the service of human development. *WHO Chronicle*, **38**(6): 239–242 (1984).

35. SADIK, N. Family planning.: improving the health of women. *Draper Fund report*, No. 9 (October 1980).

36. RUTSTEIN, S. O. *Infant and child mortality: levels, trends and demographic differentials.* Voorburg, Netherlands, International Statistical Institute and WFS, 1983 (Comparative Studies No. 24).

37. HARRISON, K. A. Child bearing, health and social priorities. A survey of 22,774 consecutive births in Zaria, Northern Nigeria. *British journal of obstetrics and gynaecology,* Supplement No. 5 (1985).

# Chapter 10

# THE CHALLENGE

---

> Primary health care has so far delivered neither sufficient care
> nor adequate health to the primary protectors of every nation's
> vitality and future health: women in their role as mothers.[1]

Often the death of a woman in childbirth signifies far more
than the tragic loss of a single life: it can threaten the
survival of the whole family. The newborn baby and other
young children who may survive her are rendered particularly
vulnerable by the loss of their mother, and research has
shown that the bereaved husband's life expectancy may also
be shortened by the death of his wife.

In most poor countries such a woman is likely to have been
the lynchpin—if not the sole supporter—of the family,
responsible for providing and preparing food, collecting
water, gathering fuelwood and looking after the children and
old people, as well, perhaps, as working outside the home for
a living. The gap that she leaves cannot easily be filled. In
one example from Kenya, the older children of three women
who died in childbirth resorted to begging in the city to
support themselves, while the children too young to fend for
themselves died (1). In another example from Ethiopia, the
three young children of a widowed woman who died in
childbirth were looked after in a casual way by her
neighbours. In the extremely poor district of the city where
they lived no one could afford to take responsibility for
orphaned children.[2]

Yet, in spite of the obviously vital role played by women in
society, their needs remain neglected, as witnessed by the
unnecessarily high levels of maternal mortality in many poor
countries. Analyses of government health budgets reveal that
many developing countries allocate less than 20% to their

---

[1] Draper, W. H. Address to Safe Motherhood International Conference, Nairobi,
1987.
[2] Kwast, B. E. *Roads to maternal health. Case histories, including comments on
preventive strategies.* World Bank Informal Paper No. 1. Safe Motherhood
International Conference, Nairobi, 10–13 February 1987.

maternal and child health programmes (MCH). Moreover, mothers are often seen primarily as vehicles for child health, so very little of the 20% allocated to MCH actually benefits the women themselves (2).

It is not easy to reach those who habitually stand silently in the shadows, but if maternal mortality rates are to be reduced, the failure of existing health services to meet the needs of most women must be recognized for what it is and action taken to alter the situation.

In most places the need is not for an expensive programme of building, equipping and staffing new facilities, but for better use to be made of buildings and personnel already in place. This requires creativity and willingness to break old moulds. It also means recognizing the often subtle barriers that exist between women and the health care system and devising services that are as sensitive as possible to the daily pattern of their lives.

It is generally agreed that within the health system, action is required on three fronts simultaneously: community-based care needs to be reassessed and strengthened; the referral facilities need to be improved; and an effective "alarm" and transport system needs to be devised to ensure that both women at risk of problems in pregnancy or labour and emergency cases can be transferred to a clinic or hospital in time for effective treatment.

But what would a programme of this nature cost? Low-income countries are currently spending around US$ 9 per head per year on health care; using data from Africa and Asia to construct realistic models, the World Bank has calculated that for an additional $ 2 per head health care for women could be strengthened to the extent of reducing maternal mortality by about 50% within a decade. Moreover, an appreciable reduction in maternal deaths could be achieved with an investment of as little as $ 1 per head (1).

Even these small sums may seem hopelessly beyond the means of some poor countries already burdened by debt and diminishing income from world trade. But it is worth noting that even the poorest countries seem able to raise funds for political struggles (3):

> In 1980 the non-oil developing countries spent over 51 billion dollars on military expenditures. Four years later the annual

spending had risen to almost 58 billion, in constant prices, a rise of over 13%. The poorest of the developing countries with a gross national product (GNP) per head in 1982 of less than US$ 400, increased their defence spending during the same period by an even higher percentage; the quantity of defence purchased by them rose in real terms by almost 21%. In the period 1980–83 the developing countries as a whole imported 65% more arms (in value terms) than they had done in the years 1976–79. And all this at a time when there was an international recession, collapse of commodity prices, decline in world trade, large scale famine, low growth and faltering development.

The purpose of raising this issue here is not to add to the controversial debate about the relationship between defence and development spending, but simply to point out that, where political will is sufficiently strong, even seemingly insurmountable obstacles can be overcome. If the case for improving maternal health care were to attract only a fraction of the political commitment to defence issues, huge progress could be made towards saving maternal lives and protecting families from the misery and insecurity occasioned by the loss of such a valuable member.

This is the challenge to both national and international leaders, and it requires a change of attitude and priorities throughout societies, from the grass roots up. A special effort to meet the needs of those who bear the greatest burden of discrimination is implicit in the call for health for all by the year 2000.

# References

1. HERZ, B. & MEASHAM, A. R. *The safe motherhood initiative: proposals for action.* Washington, DC, World Bank, 1987.
2. HOWARD, D. Aspects of maternal morbidity: the experience of developing countries. In: Jelliffe, D. B. & Jelliffe E. F. P., ed. *Advances in international maternal and child health.* Vol. 7. Oxford, Clarendon Press, 1987, pp. 1–35.
3. DEGER, S. Resource transfer from defence to health care: problems and possibilities. *Journal of tropical pediatrics*, **33** (Supplement 1): 26–33 (1987).

# INDEX

(t) = table, (f) = figure